Compassionate Recovery

Darren Littlejohn

Copyright © 2022 Darren Littlejohn
compassionaterecovery.us

Published by Rainbow Light Media, Portland, OR

Cover by germancreative

Library of Congress Control Number: 2022907918
ISBN: 978-0-9895260-4-3
Printed in The United States of America
First Edition Trade Paperback
May 2022

All rights reserved.
No portion of this book may be reproduced in any form without permission from the publisher, except as permitted by U.S. copyright law. For permissions contact:
info@compassionaterecovery.us

Although the publisher and the author have made every effort to ensure that the information in this book was correct at press time and while this publication is designed to provide accurate information in regard to the subject matter covered, the publisher and the author assume no responsibility for errors, inaccuracies, omissions, or any other inconsistencies herein and hereby disclaim any liability to any party for any loss, damage, or disruption caused by errors or omissions, whether such errors or omissions result from negligence, accident, or any other cause. This book is not intended as a substitute for the medical advice of physicians. The reader should regularly consult a physician in matters regarding their health, and with respect to any symptoms that may require diagnosis or medical attention.

For information about special discounts available for bulk purchase, sales promotions, fund-raising, and educational needs, contact the author directly at info@compassionaterecovery.us

To send a book to a prisoner, treatment center client, or armed services member, please see compassionaterecovery.us to join the Books for Addicts Campaign

Printed in the U.S.A.

Published by Rainbow Light Media
Portland OR

Part I ii
1. Our Common Humanity 9
2. Adverse Childhood Experiences (ACEs) 32
3. Effects of ACEs 52
4. ACEs and Recovery 73

Part II 103
5. The Spectrum of Stress 110
6. The Window of Tolerance 120
7. The Nervous System 131
8. Neurotransmitters 142
9. Your Brain 160
10. Your Brain on Addiction 172
11. Your Brain on Trauma 188

Part III 212
12. Your Brain on Mindfulness 214
13. Your Brain on Empathy 233
14. Your Brain on Self-compassion 245
15. Your Brain on Compassion 255

Part IV 271
16. Your Recovery, Your Way 272
17. Funnel Traps 292

18. The Recovery-Mastery Spectrum 325
19. Mastery 335
20. Practicing the Principles 351
21. Compassionate Communication 361
22. Compassionate Community 371
Conclusion 412
Additional Resources 414

Acknowledgments

Over the course of the past few years, there are many people who have helped me sustain myself. To all, thank you.

Special thanks to John McCarthy for his ongoing support over the years. My friend Robert Smith from Louisiana as well. Tysa and Amy, as always, never left my going through another book delivery. Rick Sendquist, for his ongoing years of reading, editing, and emotional support, thank you, sir. My buddy Aari @gilamonsterglass got me through some rough periods of isolation during COVID. When I had no car and needed meds, he delivered. Thank you so much.

Jean, thank you so very much.

No one helped me more than my agent, Barbara Deal, who came out of retirement to support this work. More than an agent, Barbara was a friend and spiritual mentor for more than a decade. Barbara, I hope you can hear me. Thank you, Barbara. May your light of faith shine through this work and help the people you want it to.

My editor is the best reader on a recovery book that I've ever had. This book wouldn't be what it is without you. Thank you.

Rachel Michelson has an associate's degree in Behavioral Science and an associate's degree in Psychology. Michelson studies Psychology and Child

Development at California State University Fullerton. Her current research is on Masculinity and Vulnerability. Michelson is a 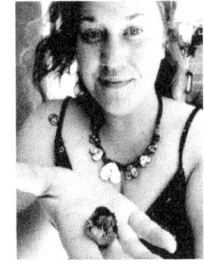 practicing shaman and has participated in a program of recovery for over a decade. She lives in Southern California. Michelson enjoys art, music, and jewelry.

Michelson can be reached at Rachel.RisingFire@gmail.com

A brilliant (and very detailed) analysis of the traumatized mind and its relationship to addictions of all kinds, and a proposed path to recovery through compassion - compassion with others, and especially with yourself. A tour de force from the author of "The 12-Step Buddhist". -Ken S.

"Darren Littlejohn presents a novel perspective to addiction recovery, based upon scientific evidence, and first-hand embodied wisdom and compassion. Compassionate Recovery is an informative guide comprised of both reasoned and intuitive tools for healing.

*To influence healing and inspire others to explore compassion within addiction recovery, he invites readers to give feedback that may be applied to future book revisions, as a living resource born from a common collective source of individuals in recovery with valuable wisdom and compassion to share."
-Susan Knier, OTD-MH, OTR/L, MBA Certified Teacher of Mindfulness and Compassion-based Interventions*

For my old dogs Zippy, Mackie, LILI, and Gizmo. And my new dogs, Gus and Moe, for teaching me what compassion really means[1].

---

[1] Dogs are the best. Save one today.

Preface

"Broadly defined, compassion is a sense of concern that arises when we are confronted with another's suffering and feel motivated to see that suffering relieved. The English word compassion, from its Latin root, literally means "to suffer with."
-Thupten Jinpa

Namaste. In yoga, we say namaste[2] as a greeting of compassion. The first time I ever heard the term was from a girl in Alcoholics Anonymous (AA) in the mid-80s. She said it meant, "the Light in me sees the Light in you." The light we talk about in this book is the Light of Compassion and its potential to heal where it hurts the most.

---

2 The term Namaste has a rich history of meaning in India. From International Journal of Medicine and Public Health 2021,11,1,63-64. DOI:10.5530/ijmedph.2021.1.12 February 2021

"'Namaste' (or 'Namaskar' or 'Namaskaram') is a common cultural verbal salutation practiced, primarily in Indian subcontinent, since ages. The term 'Namaste' has been derived from two Sanskrit words; 'namah' meaning 'bow', 'obeisance', 'adoration' or 'reverential salutation' and 'te' connotes 'to you'. And, the gesture 'Namaste' epitomizes that there is a divine spark in each ones heart chakra i.e. an salutation of ones soul by another."

Have you ever stared at candlelight for a while and felt a little focused after? When I was 22, we did this meditation in drug treatment. We sat in a dark room on a pillow with a candle in front of us. The nun who was leading the class instructed us to "Be in the now. Breathe. Become the candle." More than thirty years later, during another meditation on the sky, I realized that we're similar to candle flames. We burn for a while; then we're gone or transformed. Depending on our point of view, what we think is ourselves just isn't here, or anywhere—anymore. When or if we go to some other place or state is a question with caboodles of declaration and speculation over the course of human history.

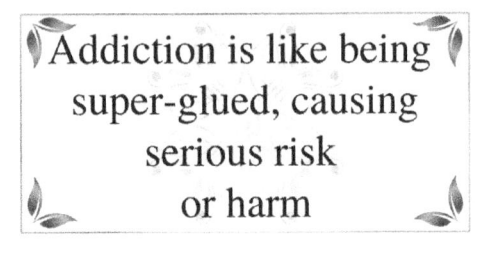

> Addiction is like being super-glued, causing serious risk or harm

First, there is a kind of darkness—we don't exist yet[3]—then some miracle creates a spark, and we become this consciousness, a kind of light. We don't know how long our light will burn. We don't generally get to know when our light will go out. Maybe we can appreciate this kind of idea on a superficial level. Most will take our temporary existence for granted until one day we're shocked to

---

[3] Buddhist teachings say there is no "I" that exists concretely. Yet simultaneously something is born.

notice that our light has ceased, probably without our permission! Then there we are—or aren't, as the case may be—sitting in the dark again.

This kind of talk can create a sense of uncertainty and impermanence, which can be unnerving. A normal response would be to reach for some kind of explanation to make sense of it all or to *make meaning*. But even if we subscribe to a great astrology newsletter, it won't ever be able to predict when our candle will flicker for the last time as the final wisp of consciousness fades into the ether. If we can come to a serious realization—a deep one that we feel in our bones—that we don't know when we'll die, we'll have an awareness that will shift every aspect of how we are in the world. At that moment,

> Attachment is a sense of being glued in unhealthy ways

we may look back and wish we'd lived more, lived better, and showed appreciation for those we care about.

Meditation on this should create a sense of urgency. Because it means we have no guarantee we'll wake up tomorrow. Neither did most of the people who didn't wake up this morning. Dying probably wasn't likely on the list. Taking this into our hearts and deeply understanding it is vital to our ability to heal. Healing involves letting go of our deepest attachment-addiction. This is part of the *why,* which says we have pretty good reason to make this effort to brighten our inner flames—while we're still able.

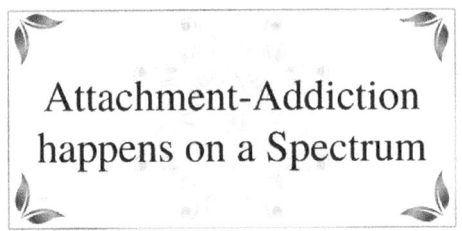

Most of us are born just bright enough. We radiate the right amount of light to get along in the world. Others may burn hot. A few blaze like brilliant stars, then disappear. Many exist in the uncertainty of a smolder—an ember that may or may not become a blaze. Those in this state may not know anything about being a "real" flame. We may feel like we have no spark at all.

If you sometimes—or often—feel this way, don't be discouraged. It's OK. Your light is still on! There's enough life force within you to spark something—perhaps an unseen potential for freedom from suffering.

Your real potential to shine *brighter than ever* is already right here, right now. It isn't somewhere else. It's not the past or future you, the recently reinvented you, nor the myriad versions of you. It's the you that's you right now, just as you are.

Let's try something to create that feeling. To tap into this, take a moment to think about your younger self, perhaps at a challenging time. Pause and consider for a moment what you would have wanted to hear most from your caregiver at that moment. What could they have said to you that would have made you feel loved?

Once you have a sense or feeling of the situation and the words you wanted to hear, put your hand on your heart, or touch your face. Close your eyes. For a moment, just feel the warmth of your precious life. As you inhale, notice the light within you glowing brighter. Now, silently or out loud, say it to your younger self. Say that thing that you wanted or needed to hear most. Be the person who has that level of compassion—for you.

Cool, you just did some self-compassion self-care. Good work. In doing so, you learned the most powerful principle this book contains. If you can feel self-compassion, that spark can become something brighter. It's there. However, if you're anything like me, it can be hard at first to feel any compassion for yourself. It took almost a year of practice for me to notice a spark, then to cultivate the flame of self-compassion—the first step in compassion for others. It is a hard thing, to be sure. You can do it. If my self-loathing self can make an inroad to internal self-acceptance, I'm confident that you can too.

In this book, you'll be introduced to concepts and skills. That will help you *discover and cultivate* the light of compassion in ways that create positive changes that will help you on the path. However, it can't be overstated that these types of personal changes will have an impact on those around you.

Considering the way things have been in the past couple of years—have always been—right now is a good time to create compassion within us to share the light with our family, work, and community. Many of the Key Takeaways are images that you can copy and use. Our working definitions and things that you need to know will be clear. In the end, you're encouraged to find your own sense of meaning and purpose, as these are suggestions to get you started.

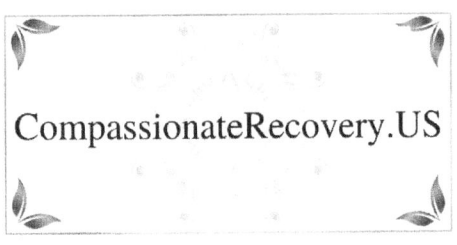

It's up to you to create your own path of recovery. Wait, you didn't know you could do that? Neither did I, but it's true. Your recovery, your way. This book is full of ideas for putting into practice the things we need to know to live a life of joy and happiness instead of pain and suffering.

Since our journey will be ongoing, the next edition of this book will need your input. This is particularly important if you're in the helping professions. All feedback is welcome, including suggested changes and new ideas for Compassionate Recovery tools. Those who've read the book and have tried some of the ideas are welcome to share feedback to feedback@compassionaterecovery.us

This book is evolving. Stay tuned for follow-up volumes. Do you want your story to be in a future edition of Compassionate Recovery? If you've been practicing the tools here and would like to share how it's changed your life, please send your story to stories@compassionaterecovery.us

Be sure to say how you'd like to be referred to; full name, first name with last initial, or professional information. All submissions will be considered and become the property of the author upon submission. You'll be entitled to a free hard copy of the next edition if your story is included.

In Compassion,
Darren Littlejohn
Gila National Forest, New Mexico
4/20/22

Compassionate Recovery

Mindful Healing for Trauma and Addictions

Darren Littlejohn

May 2022
Rainbow Light Media
Portland, OR

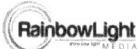

Part I

The Why

"It is possible that the next Buddha will not take the form of an individual. The next Buddha may take the form of a community—a community practicing understanding and loving kindness, a community practicing mindful living. This may be the most important thing we can do for the survival of the earth."
-Thich Nhat Hanh[4]

Whatever your dope is, welcome. Thank you for buying or stealing this book. If it's for you, keep it with you. Write in it, make notes. If you know someone who's suffering, put a copy somewhere they can accidentally find it.

Do we need another recovery book? Absofuckinloutely. In fact, despite all our efforts, addicts continue to suffer more than ever. Unfortunately, if you're reading this, it's probable that you know more than one person with problematic attachment-addiction. Maybe yourself. Dr. Sanjay Gupta reported on CNN[5] that overdoses from April 2020 to April 2021 went from 78,000 to

---

4 (2016). "The Miracle of Mindfulness, Gift Edition", p.29, Beacon Press

5 Wed December 1, 2021 CNN

https://www.cnn.com/2021/12/01/politics/fentanyl-drug-overdose-addiction-what-matters/index.html

100,000. This is an increase of 28.5%. It's clear that despite everything we've done, addiction is winning.

Something that addresses these issues from a fresh perspective has been desperately needed for a very long time. We're not reinventing the wheel. This is more like constructing a new kind of vehicle designed to take us on our journey using a combination of existing technology and some much-needed upgrades. When you begin driving, you're in charge of how fast and how far you go and the destination.

It's said in Alcoholics Anonymous that it's a *simple program for complicated people*. Compassionate Recovery is much simpler. In specialized recovery groups that focus on one aspect of addiction exclusively, alcohol, for example, it can be difficult and confusing to tease out what program treats what addiction. When I was in early recovery, I went to four or five *different* 12-Step groups to manage areas of attachment-addiction with relationships, alcohol, drugs, codependency, and emotions. The only other option was to filter what was being shared about alcohol, for example, and try to apply it to food or sex. That can be anything but simple, especially when we need to share our heart. We shouldn't have to worry about filtering. Addiction is addiction, and it happens on a spectrum that starts with hooks, called attachments. Therefore, if I'm sharing about gambling in a meeting about sex, it's unreasonable to expect to find others who can relate. The practices in this book can reduce or eliminate that sense of feeling out of place in a recovery meeting.

This guide is written to apply simply. There are no steps that must be worked with a sponsor in the order they're presented. There is no hierarchy of sponsors for newcomers [6] or old-timers with many years of recovery to people with less time.

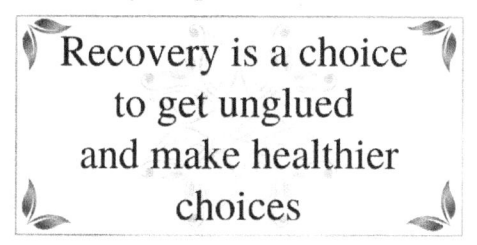

> Recovery is a choice to get unglued and make healthier choices

Compassionate Recovery adds a range of tools arranged in new ways—a kind of system without steps in a particular sequence. This book, therefore, isn't merely a new book on recovery. It's a new *kind* of book meant to be used in innovative ways. The practices in this book are designed to cut through the root of the problems of attachment-addiction that plague us relentlessly in our culture and in our own lives. Built on but utterly different from any previous works by me or others in the field of recovery. It's not a Buddhism or a Yoga book, per se. It is, however, inspired by my own experience, observation, and study as a Buddhist yogi in recovery. While this book isn't about me or my story, sharing is clarifying when necessary. In future editions, your story could be included. The original

---

6 originally called 'pigeons' by AA old timers

AA book was written by 100 people. Maybe over time, there will be others who contribute to this idea.

I'll share my personal why for doing this work. It's an essential aspect of why I *must* be on a path of healing.

The idea was evoked by the necessity to survive my personal journey. This is due to my own challenges and faith that solutions are possible. Since what I was doing was working, the ideas eventually expanded into more advanced research and studied for a much broader application. The goal is to exclude no one from this path of healing.

Another of the many compelling reasons for this book is that I intend to hold the vows that I took to help end suffering until all the beings are free of suffering. We had plenty of addiction when this project started, but there is now more suffering than ever. Isolation, depression, and anxiety are part of our conversations at the grocery check-out all over the country.

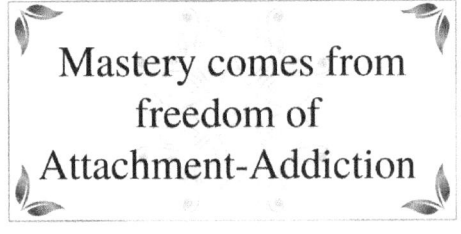

Mastery comes from freedom of Attachment-Addiction

COVID-19 and its social impact forced us to seek and find recovery in entirely new ways. We've learned new workarounds, but the limited solutions and inherent problems in most recovery models are clear to me. In recent years many great solutions for addicts have emerged.

There is so much coming to light. We finally have new thinking, which we discuss further on. We haven't seen a universal, inclusive, trauma-sensitive recovery guide that applies the salve of compassion to the core wounds where we suffer the most. Best of all, we can recover right out in the open. There's no need for the shame of anonymity. There's a more profound, internal way to practice anonymity which we discover on the path to compassion and wisdom.

I like to look for connections. You'll find some interesting correlations here. I hope the way I've chosen to organize these principles and practices will do good where it's needed. Any work that helps addicts ease suffering is wonderful and worth it. Too many friends and neighbors have died suffering in addiction. Maybe you don't have to.

Even if just one addict or their kid suffers less, the benefit is immeasurable because all beings have infinite potential to become fully liberated from the realm of suffering.[7] It makes sense that all of us have this infinite potential because time is infinite. There is no known beginning, so how can there be an end? In infinite time there is infinite possibility. We endlessly cycle through our rebirths due to our attachments in this and many lives. The cycle of addiction, which is the nature of suffering, can be broken. Not just duct-taped and patched together *good enough for government work,* as my dad used to

---

[7] Known in Tibetan Buddhism as a Perfectly Completed Buddha or Awakened One.

say. The cycle of suffering can be broken. Liberation is not only possible but also our Divine responsibility to develop our own unique expression.

A big part of my *why* is people like my friend Mary, an intelligent, attractive, and kind 30-year-old who worked at a high-level technical job. She had an amazing, loving family. When she drank and drugged, bad things happened. Despite years of trying to recover in all the usual ways, she wound up drunk over and over. She eventually spiraled into crystal meth use and sought higher levels of stimulation in a bizarre underground sex culture—not the kind based on healthy practices. My beautiful friend got in a car at a dive bar with a whacked-out couple and their buddy. She was later killed and dumped in a nearby park.

I had her little dog, Jimmy, for many years after that. He passed right before COVID-19 hit. When he looked at me with those massive Shi-tzu eyes, I often told him, "Your momma loves you and asked me to take care of you, and that's what I'm gonna do!" I still miss them. I wish I could have done more and done better. This book is partly a response to watching this pattern with countless suffering addicts for too many years.

Compassionate Recovery can help members of our communities. Nearly everybody's lost someone to severe addiction. I have more in common with Mary than many on a traditional path of recovery. Like me, she never felt understood in traditional 12-Step programs. It was difficult, but I was able to deal with this sense of not being in the right place in meetings. I've maintained my recovery, but many don't. We tried all the tools available, including the alternative style 12-Step Buddhist groups that we had at the Portland Zen Center for many years. That program was created because it was the kind of community where I felt comfortable. Ultimately, though, it wasn't entirely right because many people don't always want to commit to a system derived from another culture.

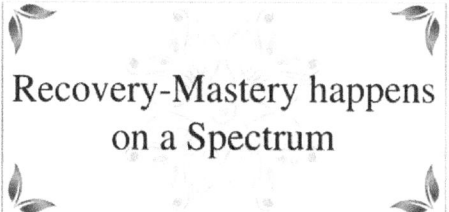

Recovery-Mastery happens on a Spectrum

The ideas of my earlier work needed to be expanded to reach more people. Unfortunately for my friend, what was needed wasn't yet available—a path of recovery that got to the root of the problem.

What is needed is a way of being in recovery that's open and inclusive to all kinds of people who may be anywhere on the attachment-addiction spectrum. At the beginning of recovery, we don't often realize how difficult the path ahead can be. It's vital to know a wide range of possibilities and ways to prevent, navigate and repair as we learn and grow on our path. It's often said in recovery that if we knew how hard it was going to be, we might not have started. I want to tell you how hard but necessary this work is so that you're equipped for the journey as you head out on the highway.

The Roadmap of Recovery that we talk about here takes a bird's eye view of known pitfalls and emphasizes ways to make new opportunities for wisdom and compassion. There's a reason for an eye toward the long-term view. I was never a Boy Scout, but I think they had a motto about being prepared. It's good to be prepared. The fewer surprises, the better. There will always be unavoidable twists and turns, but our road trip will be smoother if we know where they are and how to deal with them.

You wouldn't climb Mt. Everest without your map, gear, and Sherpa, right? You would have done your research. The fact that there are bodies up there on the ice is not lost on you.

If we can conceptualize the path of recovery in terms of spectrums, it can increase mindfulness of one of the most important principles of this book: our common humanity. We're not so different. There's more in common that connects us than separates us. Everyone is simultaneously in various stages of growth on many different spectrums. We all have myriad aspects of "selves" that exist in their own ways in the spectrums of attachment-addiction or recovery-mastery. The whole of our existence is moving and dynamic. We can be in different places on our various dimensions one day and others the next.

The recovery-mastery spectrum is a framework for healing that gives you the space to grow your recovery your way. It's not necessary to fit a square peg in a round hole. Be you, wherever you are in any aspect, anywhere, you find yourself.

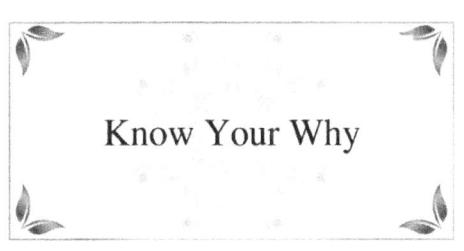

We are all in unique, changing places on multiple spectrums of experience. There are many dimensions of complexity in our human experience. Let's condense our focus to the physical, emotional, mental, and spiritual[8] dimensions for clarity.

Practice:
What's your why?

Write down your first thoughts.

---

[8] These are presented in order of most concrete, tangible and measurability. You can see and feel your height and weight, but it's harder to measure your spiritual experience.

Chapter 1
Our Common Humanity

"Sun is up, I'm a mess
Gotta get out now, gotta run from this
Here comes the shame, here comes the shame
1, 2, 3, 1, 2, 3 drink
1, 2, 3, 1, 2, 3 drink
1, 2, 3, 1, 2, 3 drink
Throw 'em back till I lose count"
-Sia[9]

The easiest way to practice compassion is to understand our common humanity or the things that make us all human. All sentient beings have sentience or consciousness in common. All humans have quite a bit more in common than not. What about those 'different' people? Easy, celebrate diversity! It's compassionate. It's fun.

Since it's great to know how we're the same and that it doesn't matter if we're different, we now have all the logic we need to practice compassion. Let's look at some basic, indisputable facts of common humanity. We can try to tell ourselves stories about

---
9 Writer(s): Furler Sia Kate I, Shatkin Jesse Samuel

how different people are due to their gender identification, race, and so forth. Still, there are many ways to find what humanness we have in common, even before we engage that human in meaningful conversation with good eye contact, listening skills and validations we know for sure that we have four dimensions in common; physical, emotional, mental, and spiritual. Exploration of these can go in any direction and are endless. Let's meditate on them briefly, as they are the basis for a lifetime of healing practice.

Physical Humanity

The most concrete and tangible domain or dimension of the human experience is our physicality. There are too many aspects of the physical body to name. We can meditate on anything that we feel from any sense that our body perceives. Regardless of who we are, everyone has something in common: to date, the perfect human has not yet been discovered. Whether we have one leg that's longer or an allergy to whiskey, our physical aspects change in different ways and at their own rates. Some of which we can influence, others we can't.

The wisdom to change the things we can tell us what we need to know so we can accept the things we cannot change because we know the difference. We can change more physical aspects now than ever before, means and resources notwithstanding.

Strength is an aspect on the physical dimension that has a spectrum. For example, upper body strength is on a different spectrum than glute power. The importance of thinking about these things is to understand that we're not all one thing or another. We're not all bad or all good. We're not real addicts or non-addicts. Instead, we're beings made up of the same stuff, arranged in similar ways on similar spectrums. Isn't that fascinating?

Drop into Dropping in

In some healing circles, the term 'dropping in' is used to describe the ability to connect with ourselves in deep and meaningful ways to our journey. Rather than merely go through the motions of understanding the material here, we need to learn skills on how to Drop into a calm state. There are as many doorways to drop in as there are moments in a day. We can enter them through our mental, physical, emotional, and spiritual dimensions.

Throughout the book, we'll drop into practices that will help us feel it so that we can heal it. There are some rules for the road that shamans use to guide participants in healing ceremonies.

The first rule is to relax. Compassion arises easier in a calm state. Let your body get still, and your mind can chill. That's numero-don't-forget-it-uno.

Another rule is that once you set off on the journey with your intentions, you need to follow the signs. You're opening up to healing energies that you need to let guide you. You can set the intention, but the rule is to follow wherever our wisdom teachers lead us. Be brave. Ask the right questions and be ready for the real answers.

If the buried stuff were easy to access and release, we wouldn't be having this conversation. When we do the work, out comes the dirt. As my mother would say, "and there are no two ways about it!"

Dropping in: Where are My Feet?

Close your eyes. Be still. Don't move a muscle. Give yourself sufficient time to drop into stillness. Then when you're as still as can be, ask yourself, "Where are my feet?" Resist the urge to wiggle your toes or shift your feet. If you wiggle, you must start over! Repeat as necessary to remember where your feet are always.

Emotional Humanity

Let's use one of our many emotions as an example: anger. We may find ourselves in a relative comfort zone regarding our ability to experience anger. Think of the range of possibilities as something like a number line, with 0 as a baseline comfort zone. On the minus side of the line, there's less and less outward anger energy to the point of depression. At the extreme of the other end, we find rage.

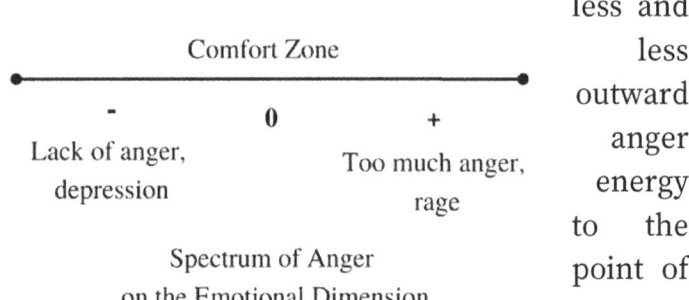

Spectrum of Anger on the Emotional Dimension

Where we are on the spectrum of anger at any given moment is dynamic, not static. It changes as we change in any situation on the spectrum of our lives. Most people don't ever experience the whole range in any spectrum. Some people are rarely angry, and others seem to be upset about something all the time. But here's the common humanity. Everyone has an emotional dimension with many aspects. No one is exempt from the emotional aspect of anger. We're all somewhere on the same continuum in this human experience that is common to all people.

We can empathize with each other because we know how it feels to be on that spectrum, even if it's not as high or low. Most people on the Earth are going to be on that spectrum somewhere. We're not outside the anger zone; we're just in a different place at a different time.

The commonness of our humanity is so easy to see everywhere if we open our eyes. We can train ourselves to look for it and live by it. This is part of the intention of Compassionate Recovery as a set of principles and practices. I return to this point periodically because this approach often leaves people asking, but what is it? It's what you want to make of it. Hopefully, there is enough material to keep you busy wherever you may find yourself on any given day in any given spectrum.

Drop into the Comfort Zone

Using the simple graph idea above, choose your top three strongest emotions that you find challenging to manage. What are some examples of when you were feeling balanced and calm about each one? What are some times that you were over the top or way down under that baseline? Write in the Notes section about what your Comfort Zones are or how you'd like them to be around your three strongest emotions. You can use fear, anger, and apathy as a quick start.

Mental Humanity

I don't know about you, but my thoughts can range from none to an Information Superhighway mental gridlock. It's impossible to stop them all. But we can notice the array of thought traffic as if a light show in the sky, just shimmering, disappearing. Nothing real or substantial. Just energy.

The mental dimension is everything that makes up our mind-space. Our thought patterns on different topics include our personality traits, linguistic abilities, communication, and problem-solving skills. Creative processes are also aspects of the mental dimension.

Memory is an excellent example of a mental aspect. Consider an event in your life, like your 16th birthday. If you try to remember every detail without the gift of a photographic memory, it might be small. Your memory spectrum of that day might be quite vivid and clear about what you felt and saw but less salient on what you heard or tasted.

Dropping in with Mind Maps

There are a number of mind maps in this book. I first learned how to make these in grad school from my thesis advisor. He was a Decision Map analyst. The maps we used were to facilitate the making of complex decisions. Don't worry. You don't need advanced statistics to make a mind map. What you need to know is that it's a powerful tool for understanding the relationships between ideas.

Find a free mind mapping app or site. I used simplemind.[10] Create a mind map of your mental "Office Space." Start in the center with who you are but use something besides your name to describe yourself. Be creative. Draw lines out to bubbles or squares that are connected, and represent aspects of you or ideas that you find important.

There is no right or wrong to this exercise. You can do it as many times and on as many ideas as you want. It's a tool for your mind to understand itself.

Spiritual Humanity

We'll go into more detail here to address some of the issues about spirituality from the start so that it doesn't get in the way as you follow this guide. Most of us can agree on what the physical, emotional, and mental dimensions are. However, when it comes to spirituality, the ice walls can go up for some of us. They can be melted away with the Light of Compassion.

What does it mean to be spiritual? Why do some have problems with the idea? The main problem that some have with the idea of spirituality is simple. The reason is trauma around religion. In 35 years in the recovery field, I've heard that people shut themselves off from the healing power of spirituality because of bad experiences with religious and

---

10 https://simplemind.eu/download/free-edition/

authority figures, including parents, clergy, and institutions.

I've seen the best results when recovering people can learn to separate experiences and biases with religion from the openness and flexibility of spirituality. Religions are often—not always—about control and dogma. This is always a hot topic. It's easy to get people to jump up and down about religion. But if you want to benefit from the total efforts of all the work on the human soul and psyche, you can't ignore religion. It is there to make things better, no matter how badly people mess it up. But the good news is that there is a way to understand the key points of various religions without converting to them or being involved any more than we want to be.

We work with principles that affect all dimensions of our lives; physical, emotional, and mental. Think of the spiritual as the global integration of all of these.

Spirituality is about being alive, whole, and free. It's not about following something or being told what to do by an institution. It's about looking within and using discipline to train your own mind. We work with principles rather than institutions. We do practices without getting bogged down in dogma. That said, we do need always to pay respect to traditional ways. A good way to practice is to be open and respectful because we don't know everything!

An artist taps deep into their soul to create poetry, music, or paintings but may be a devout atheist. They're still doing spiritual work. The spirit is the mystery, the unseen forces. No one knows where we came from, how we got here, or where we're going. Science, art, philosophy, *and* religion try to answer these questions. But they're also questions that can be dealt with in simple terms by practicing the Core Principles of Compassion.

We can practice spirituality within the confines of a strict religious system. Or we can practice it outside of any system. We have total freedom in our choices regarding how we approach our healing and development. If we're in groups, the members should be supportive and respectful about each other's journey regardless of conflicts or superficial differences. Compassionate Recovery is about practicing compassion with equanimity for ourselves and others, even if conflicts are interpersonal or intrapersonal (between aspects of ourselves).

To ultimately deal with addiction at its core, in addition to science, we can turn to the most powerful and ancient tools known to humanity that are spiritual in nature. These systems, such as Metaphysical Christianity, Buddhism, Yoga, Western esotericism, and others, offer paths beyond mere abstinence—to a life of fulfillment and joy. Some provide permanent salvation in one form or another. But we'll never get there if we're dead from addiction. Compassionate Recovery focuses on getting soberfrom things on the spectrum, staying sober, and thriving. From there, we can evolve to higher levels. The world needs this right now. If we take this work seriously, we can make substantial changes for ourselves and our communities.

The endpoint of addiction is death. The endpoint of Compassionate Recovery is freedom from suffering. Empower yourself to use any tool that makes sense to you. Use this framework to give you a way to see the bigger picture. That can be a roadmap to take you from where you don't want to be to where you do want to be. These maps can and will be modified as we go. Reality is dynamic. We're learning more all the time. Nothing is carved in stone. Be open. Be flexible. Be fluid. That's pretty spiritual.

Drop into Compassion as a Higher Power

Sit for a while. Be still and mindful. Reflect on the experience you're having right now in your body. Are you feeling anything emotionally? Where is it in your body? Notice your thoughts as if you are walking into a packed movie theater midway. You're not stuck in it like the audience. Read the following meditation. Pause to consider any feelings it may arouse as you read. Come back to this often. Write about it after each practice session.

Compassion is the higher power, not some deity in the sky. It's not somewhere else. It's not someone else. Compassion is your own being. Compassion is the being of all beings—the heart of all beings and the heart of all Wisdom.

The deity is your own Wisdom. If I see someone suffering on the side of the road, do they have to pray to me and beg me to help them? No. From the heart of compassion, I spontaneously help them because I know the truth of my own suffering. This is our shared humanity. This is the truth of compassion and Wisdom. There are higher beings than us, just like we're higher beings to small animals and children. Those beings, be they part of ourselves-or other souls, who are stronger and more evolved-can help us. But as collaborators, not egomaniacal gods. We just need to tap into the energy of compassion within ourselves and know that it is the same at the heart of all beings, big and small.

This means it's time to own your own magnificence. It's possible to accept your birthright as heir to the kingdom without becoming addicted to power like some crazy king.

This is the truth of suffering. This is the Wisdom of compassion. May we own our own power without being addicted to it. That power is compassion. That power makes it possible to love ourselves and each other like a mother loves her only child.

In the spiritual domain, it's difficult to measure degrees on a spectrum separate from other dimensions. We might have had some spiritual experiences or feel like we've had none at all yet. If we simply consider the spiritual as the non-material, it's clear that everything in our experience is spiritual. That's because spirituality, even if it's from a higher dimension is still experienced through the physical, emotional, and mental dimensions. There is a point of spiritual mastery that profound spiritual teachings lead to that is a state beyond what is known as the three gates of the body, speech (energy), and mind to a knowledge equivalent to spiritual mastery, but we're not going there right now.

We experience, interpret, and analyze the world through our five senses. Think about it. How would you get any information about the universe if you had no sense of sight, smell, taste, touch, or sound? Some behaviorists say anything extra-sensory or beyond the senses, such as a spiritual feeling, is pure imagination.

Yet somehow, we have something of a sixth sense, a global or intuitive way to know things. It's not material or directly related to the senses, but it can't be separated from the senses. Does that make sense? It's possible to create spiritual feelings and experiences through practice. We can then integrate the wisdom gained into our sober skill set. Sometimes ordinary experiences are illuminated in a spiritual way. For example, the tactile sensation of a kiss will be the same raw physical experience whoever the lucky recipient might be. But if it's someone special, we get a spiritual feeling. It's part emotional feeling, part physical experience, and part mental story.

An example of an aspect on the spiritual dimension is an interest in spiritual matters. On the radical left (-0) on the spectrum, we would have no spiritual interest at all. The middle (1) baseline comfort zone would be a feeling of contentment in our path. At the end of the spectrum (∞) is a level of mastery.

Another aspect that's easy to measure is the spectrum of joy. If you're anything like me, there is no memory of a joyous experience in my life. My spectrum of joy begins at minus zero. To move up the spectrum toward the light is working on a single dimension of myself (spiritual) on a single spectrum (joy). That's a specific focus on a particular area of growth that I wanted to develop after conducting a retreat on it. It took a lot of work, but I learned how to settle down my trauma responses enough to cultivate some joy. You can too.

We, humans, are on common ground on many dimensions and spectrums. There aren't many people walking around totally free of problematic attachment-addiction. We have more in common than we might think if we let go of our inner conspiracy theories about how they're out to get us. When we look at the other person and know we're on common ground, there's much less need for a defense or an offense.

If we feed on the news and scarf down the nightly rhetoric, we might not realize that our neighbor is also a dog lover who likes to BBQ, even though some of our closely held beliefs are polar opposites. Go figure. We can still break bread.[11] Look for the similarities!

Seek out things that make you and the other person human. That's what you have in common. Connect on those things. The principle at hand is called common humanity. When we practice it, we can connect with other human beings on wonderful new levels.

It's easy to be attracted to Esoteric Wisdom Traditions and Eastern spiritual teachings that have an allure. But we're often surprised at how difficult the work is once we get down to it. Thinking we might find greener grass, we buzz around like a honeybee, sniffing this and that Marigold or that Calendula. Eventually, if we want to learn something, we need to commit to a consistent path. But the path doesn't mean the focus has to be limited to one specific support group dealing with one type of attachment or addiction. No one-size-fits-all

---

11 Or a gluten free substitute!

approach works, just like no one pill that cures all ills. We need an integrated approach.

We tend to want to stick with our own so that we feel at home. From the perspective of Compassionate Recovery, there's no need for different groups with different addictions or beliefs, sexual preferences, gender identifications, or economic statuses. There's no reason *not* to go to as few or as many groups or programs that we choose. There is no rule about how it must be done, in what order, or on what timeline. The work will be there, and it will present itself to you in the way you need it to unfold. The door of recovery based on principles and practices of compassion is always open and ready when you are.

Many attempts have been made to reinvent recovery and add new cures. Most of the time, these fade away, but some stick. Usually, they're a form of 12-Step. But things are changing, which we discuss in detail.

People on the attachment-addiction spectrum need a book to be accessible yet challenging to break through the bullshit that we drop on our path. We tend to poop all over the place and then get mad at someone else when we step in it. If you're looking for sugar coating, you won't find it here.

We need an approach that serves as a contemporary guide that stays current. Imagine a book that isn't a hundred years old to help us on our path of healing. Due to book publishing technology these days, this book can instantly be updated and thus kept current. All it takes is an upload. This wasn't available in the 1930s when the first AA book was published. We can easily keep things up to date now. Remember, send in your suggestions any time. Everything will be read and considered.

Because of the pervasive suffering caused by attachment-addiction, we need a book that anyone can use. It must contain the original potency of the principles on which it is based, whatever their origin—but that people don't feel weird about. It is true that the ideas in some non-Western systems can seem odd to us at first. It's because they're different from what we grew up with. To benefit, we need a way to open up to these powerful ideas without the obstacles of understanding that can happen when we buy hook, line, and sinker to a group or organization. That's what the aim is here. Principles before memberships!

The in-group/out-group drive, while functional in many respects, continues to be a major problem. It's been exacerbated by social media and other chaotic forces. The issue is well studied in Social Psychology, Sociology and Anthropology. This tribal separation has been with Homo Sapiens since civilization began. Banding together is a human survival tool. Treating everyone with Compassionate Equanimity is a next-level survival tool. What used to be us vs. them evolves. It becomes just...us.

If you learn this tool, you'll have something of high value to offer any and all beings that you encounter. This book's foundational principle that we can practice and apply with the warring aspects of ourselves and between "us and them."

Buddha, for example, didn't have social media and pandemic chaos diluting his message. A lot of the wisdom gets lost, convoluted, and misappropriated over time. Just look at the bizarro-world misinformation campaigns and how successful they can be.

Here are some facts that are the real why behind Compassionate Recovery. How many addicts would you guess die in a year? Close your eyes and pick a number! We started the why with some stats. Let's keep in mind the level and scope of suffering that attachment-addiction causes.

In 2018 there were 67,637[12] drug overdose deaths reported in the US alone. That's not all drugs, just the most common ones. In a year, there are 8760 hours. That means that every hour in the US, something like eight addicts die. The actual number would be much higher if we had the data to include all drugs. You get the point. We need to do more. We can and should do better. We need this now more than ever.

---

[12] drugabuse.gov

Integration Practice

What's your why? It can be any number of reasons but get to the one(s) that will carry you through when it gets rough. It's going to get rough. You need your why in your back pocket the same way you have a spare tire in your car.

Write down the first impressions, ideas, feelings, or ideas that come up for you right now. This is an ongoing life practice. Check your why and walk that talk. Integrate your why into your heart, so you feel it with you all the time. Find the why that drives you.

Talk about your why in as much detail as you wish in whatever format is interesting and fun. Here's a little space. You're encouraged to keep a journal for long-term practice.

a little space

If words aren't coming to you, it's OK. Start where you are! Even if your thoughts are flowing fine, it's good to take a meditation break. How it is in this moment is fine. Let's just get a little information about how it is right now in your body. Sit still. Breathe slow and easy. From a more relaxed place, try to get a sense of your why as if it lives somewhere in your body. Where would it be? Can you gently place your loving hand of compassion there? If difficult feelings come up, try to stay with them. Just be present. Don't push. It's OK to chill. Come back later. Or just breathe.

Be brave. Ask your body what's at the core of this attachment-addiction. This is an ongoing personal inventory. Learn to ask, "Where do I need to heal the most?" Learn compassionate presence with yourself. To touch these raw nerves is painful. But we must in order to heal because this is what drives our compulsions. Feeling feelings is hard. To be numb is worse. It's important to acquire the skill of embodying the feelings, memories, or experiences that caused suffering and can now lead you toward a path of healing. But it may take time and support.

A therapist who is skilled in trauma and addiction approaches can help. There are somatic (body-oriented) therapies and movement practices that can support you in integrating rather than avoiding the roots of what causes us to suffer.

Over time, people who practice healthy brain healing in recovery are open to and explore any activity that enhances and deepens the desire for recovery. See yourself from many different angles. Ask others for feedback. Invite them to join you in recovery fun days where you can act, paint, dance, sing, climb rocks, or be of service in any way that lets you be all about your why. Try different things. If you already have a thing, try a new thing. New actions get new results. These energetic shifts move stuff around inside you. The plan is to find something to do—however regular makes sense—

that helps you see your experiences from new perspectives.

The importance of knowing your why cannot be overstated. If it's not clear, don't panic. As they say in 12-Step, more will be revealed.

Notes

Chapter 2
Adverse Childhood Experiences (ACEs)

"What matters is that you show the children, with your time and attention, that you believe in them, and that they have worth, that they can do hard things, and that you love them.[13]"

-Ben Affleck

On January 15th, 1995, the Dallas Cowboys had a debilitating break in their Superbowl streak when they lost the NFC Championship 28-38 to our Bay Area heroes, the San Francisco 49ers. Steve Young outpassed the legendary Troy Aikman, and the 49ers went on to win the Superbowl 49-26 against San Diego.

I'd moved to Texas from Long Beach, where I was finishing up my master's on the way to a Ph.D. It felt like the right thing to do, as decisions in the state of hyperarousal during a manic episode can. But I didn't have the knowledge of my condition at that time that I do now. No one did. The science wasn't available yet.

---

[13] on Howard Stern, December 14, 2021

Now, if you know anything about Texas, you know there is nothing more important than their Cowboys. This is more than a sport. It's an obsession and a cultural identity that's just part of the fabric.

As you can imagine, the next morning in downtown Dallas you could hear a pin drop. There was almost no movement, like a scene from a sci-fi post-apocalypse moment. In a new Jerry Garcia silk tie, I stood outside KDFW-TV 4, secretly quivering with joy as I huffed down a Marlboro red. In a few moments, I'd be rushing in to meet the madmen of Fox News who were taking over our CBS station. "Keep doing your jobs as normal," they said. If you ever hear that, run.

A novice number cruncher, I provided Nielsen data to the sales staff. They survived on selling "spots," 10, 20, 30-second ads that ran between syndicated reruns, or if they really wanted to spend money, the CBS Evening News offered a high market share and about 2 million viewers. Spots were sold based on ratings and market share. The job was to give them the ratings breakdowns which they used to sell advertising for the station. Nowadays, a Tik-Tok teenager has 80M followers, which is interesting considering they fired me for talking about the Internet too much. In fact, I built the station's first news website. Not bitter. They didn't quite see the value at the time.

Young, dumb, and full of myself, I finally felt cool. I had all the typical things that are supposed to make you feel good; an alright car, a decent house, and a cool job working in television. Then one day, the new General Manager introduced himself as a "guerilla marketer" when he took over our station. As CBS, the station was a staple for the 54+ white male demographic for decades in the Dallas/Ft. Worth market. They played Matlock, Dallas, and Golden. These Fox hotshots came with their 18-25 oriented programming like The Simpsons and Married with Children.

They brought in a heavy hitter General Manager of News. Let me give you an idea of how much he liked me. I piped up during the sales meetings with creative ideas on how to take advantage of the upcoming Internet revolution in the news. The response? He said, "Darren, you sound like you're on bad mushrooms. Let's not talk about the Internet anymore. Nobody knows what's going to happen." My ideas would prove useful to every news agency on the planet in the following years. Alas, a California psychedelic twenty-something trying to swim in the same water as those barracudas was doomed from Day One.

The air was warm and dank in Lower Greenville, and I really wanted to forget about the stress at work. My co-workers and I were worried about our jobs and wanted to blow off steam. We went out to a seedy bar called "Club One," where a lot of very druggy and sexy things went on in an Ecstasy-filled, cash-fueled yuppie environment where the bass was meant to jiggle your guts.

Kathy was one of the old CBS producers trying to keep my head off the chopping block. She was unsuccessful at that. But she did turn me on to MDMA, which ended a ten-year run of sobriety for me. That was my last night out in the clubs and the beginning of a very bad run that left me high and dry in the most literal of ways. But people like me with high ACEs are prone to such drama as we replay our traumas from childhood. My ACEs were high, and so was I.

Have you ever lost all your shit? I mean, like people who've been in a fire or a hurricane lose all their shit. Well, this was one of the many times that a bipolar addict like me lost his shit and his possessions. Dallas is not a cool place to relapse for a smart-ass California kid. Not recommended. I wound up on a circuitous route back to sobriety. On December 4th, 1997, I took my last drink of alcohol. I had to go back to AA because it was really the only game in town back then. Yet I always knew it left many unanswered questions, which ate at me as I sat in meetings year after year. I was doing the work but still unable to be in my body.

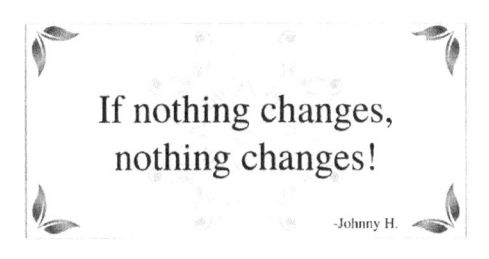

> If nothing changes, nothing changes!
> -Johnny H.

Twenty years later, long into my AA sobriety again, I remembered something from a blackout decades before. In a moment of clarity, I remembered a drunken, drug-crazed night with a guy named Luke. He was a cool club guy who wore all black and knew where to get stuff. I remembered that he snatched the glasses off my face and threw them out the window, over the fence, into the neighbor's yard for no apparent reason. I was so fucked up and blacked out that I didn't even know what had happened to my glasses. When I woke up in a hangover and Vicodin-filled haze the following evening, I didn't know where my glasses were.

I'd spent my money at the clubs, so there was no way to get new glasses. Things spiraled from there. I lost my computer job since I couldn't see the screen. But all of this was so many years past. I was sober for decades. Yet, this trauma must have been recorded deep in the part of the brain that stores traumatic memories.[14] Yet I didn't recall it for over twenty years, and it just popped into my head. An addict can get into this kind of nonsense after a decade of sobriety, step work, and spiritual development. How could this have happened to me when I did all the things they told me to do to grow up and be a sober, responsible member of society?

I did tons of therapy—thousands of meetings. Yet the *why* was never answered regarding how this

---

14 We'll cover some brain basics in an upcoming chapter.

relapse could have blindsided a nice sober guy like me. My whole life unraveled in just a few months, and it seemed to come out of nowhere. It didn't, there was a pattern and a process, but I wouldn't know that without many more years of suffering.

The Texas experience—my big move and big idea—was like getting rammed in the head by one of them steer horns they put on the grills of their Lincoln Continentals down there in Texas. They had their own ideas about big. I lost the job, the house, custody of my son, my dignity, and a bunch more stuff. I walked away with a backpack and went to a treatment center that was supposed to help me understand why I relapsed with ten years of good AA work. It didn't answer those questions, but it did get me on track to understanding how my childhood trauma affected me. They didn't really have much to offer as a solution long-term besides medication and 12-Step. More of the same wasn't going to get to the core of the problem for me. I sat there staring at the wall because there were two choices--backward or forward. But it seemed that going forward wasn't going to take me anywhere new. Something drastic was needed, but I didn't know what. One thing I knew for sure was that if nothing changes, nothing changes.

My training in Graduate Psychology included work in treatment centers and psych units. The programs were about controlling behavior, changing thought patterns, and taking tons of medication. Maybe they were helpful to some people, but the approach doesn't work for the far end of the spectrum—serious addiction. In 12-Step, the answer was always the same. Go to meetings. Help others. Don't drink in between meetings. Nothing prepared me for the relapse, and nothing could have convinced me to get sober again if I'd known how much suffering I'd encounter, even stone-cold sober. For some of us, when we stop indulging in the objects of our attachment, the experience seems intolerable. But it isn't. We can tolerate it, and we can heal.

Maybe you've known people like me. Perhaps you're one of us. Or a spouse, family member, or friend from school. We're everywhere. We're the people you cannot understand why, regardless of progress, they always dive right back into the cesspool of addiction.

During this time, when I was back into deep addiction, Dr. Vincent Felliti, who was chief of Kaiser Permanente's Department of Preventive Medicine in San Diego, was about to stumble on the answer for many of us on the spectrum of attachment-addiction. Unfortunately, it would be nearly 25 years before the picture would apply to attachment-addiction.

The ACEs Story

Dr. Felitti had worked on obesity programs at Kaiser Permanente in San Diego since the mid-80s, but in 1995 they came across an unexpected finding. They didn't know it, but their work would eventually shed some light on how some of us find sobriety intolerable. For whatever reason, no matter how hard we tried, we couldn't get comfortable in our own skin.

They were trying to understand why people could lose weight with their obesity programs, but they always put it back on. Patients could regularly lose the weight—as high as 600 lbs.—but the program didn't get to the root cause. They would inevitably put every bit of the weight back on and then some. The team felt it necessary to learn how people could stay healthy.

To understand their weight as it related to childhood development, Felliti started asking different questions, such as how much they weighed at pivotal moments in their lives.

"How much did you weigh when you were first sexually active?" and questions like it revealed that a significant majority of the obese patients had been sexually abused by adults in childhood. There was a connection between these events and the onset of weight gain. But it needed to be explored further with more subjects.

Here's a shocker. When he presented the data at research conferences, Dr. Felitti was shut down by his colleagues.[15] They felt self-reporting couldn't be trusted and recommended he get more subjects to run a more extensive study. However, Dr. Felitti was not to be dissuaded, for which we can be forever grateful! Luckily, he was able to find another researcher who was equally committed to understanding this phenomenon.

Dr. Robert Anda, an epidemiologist whose current database holds more than 200 publications to his credit, worked at the Centers for Disease Control and Prevention in Atlanta. According to his website[16], Dr. Anda conducted research in disease surveillance, behavioral health, mental health and disease, cardiovascular disease, psychosocial origins of health-risk behaviors, and childhood determinants of health. He was passionate about the same issues as Dr. Felitti.

They teamed up, which made the following discoveries possible. Because of the number of people coming through Kaiser-Permanente, they could add enough subjects to the study to convince any skeptics.

"In two waves, Felitti and Anda asked 26,000 people who came through the department "if they would be interested in helping us understand how

---

15 Today we might call them reality deniers in a male dominated structure of intrinsic abuse of power on women, LBGTQ, black, brown, Asian humans.

16 https://www.aceinterface.com/Robert_Anda.html

childhood events might affect adult health," says Felitti. Of those, 17,421 agreed."[17]

The study, known as the CDC-Kaiser Permanente Adverse Childhood Experiences (ACE) Study,[18] is one of the chief scientific inquiries into childhood abuse, neglect, and other challenges and their impact on long-term health and well-being into adulthood.

The team collected a staggering amount of data that blasted open the lens of understanding—as it does for most of us who learn about this for the first time—by looking back into adverse childhood experiences. The study also opened the field to studying the effects of traumatic experiences—short or long—far into adulthood.

With such irrefutable numbers, the results of their study were then taken seriously. In fact, they created a new knowledge base on a wide range of other health problems, among them addiction.

The ACE survey questions were based on ten *categories*, not instances of childhood trauma. For every category of trauma experienced, a single point is given to the ACE score. If there were multiple occurrences of physical abuse, one point is given for experiencing that category of abuse. If you have

---

17 From acestoohigh.com, an excellent resource.

18 "The original ACE Study was conducted at Kaiser Permanente from 1995 to 1997 with two waves of data collection. Over 17,000 Health Maintenance Organization members from Southern California receiving physical exams completed confidential surveys regarding their childhood experiences and current health status and behaviors"

https://www.cdc.gov/violenceprevention/childabuseandneglect/acestudy/about.html

both an alcoholic parent and a sibling with mental illness, your ACE score would be two because those are two categories of adverse experiences.

ACES don't happen as isolated events. If one category was experienced, there was an 87% chance of having at least one other category in the subject's past. Women were 50% more likely to have experienced *five or more* categories of childhood trauma.

Abuse
Physical – beating, not spanking (28%)

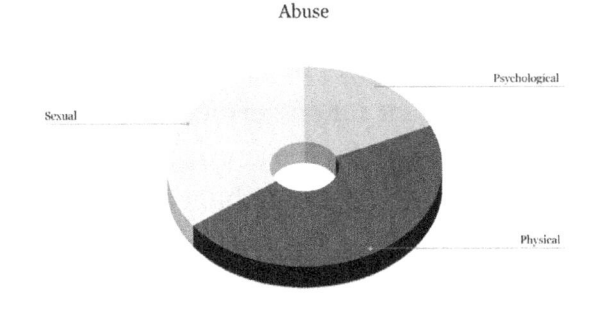

Abuse

Psychological\Emotional – recurrent threats, humiliation (11%)
Sexual – contact sexual abuse (22%, 28% women, 16% men)

Neglect
Physical (60%)
Emotional (40%)

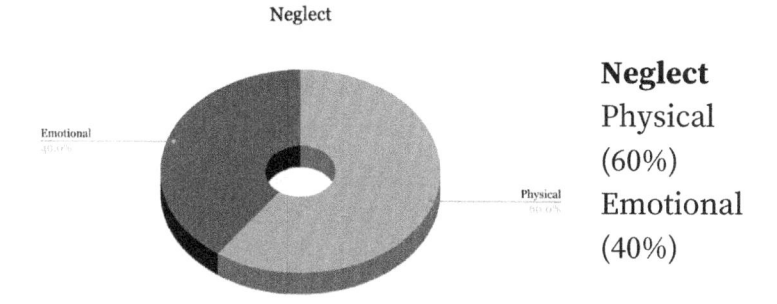

Household Challenges\Dysfunction

a parent who's an alcoholic or drug user (27%)
a mother who's a victim of domestic violence (13%)
a family member in jail\criminal behavior (6%)
a family member chronically depressed, suicidal, mentally ill, or in a psychiatric hospital (17%)
parental separation; the disappearance of a parent through divorce, death, or abandonment (23%)[19]

---

19 Lanius, R., Vermetten, E., & Pain, C. (Eds.). (2010). The Impact of Early Life Trauma on Health and Disease: The Hidden Epidemic. Cambridge: Cambridge University Press, Chapter 8. doi:10.1017/CBO9780511777042

ACEs (circular diagram)

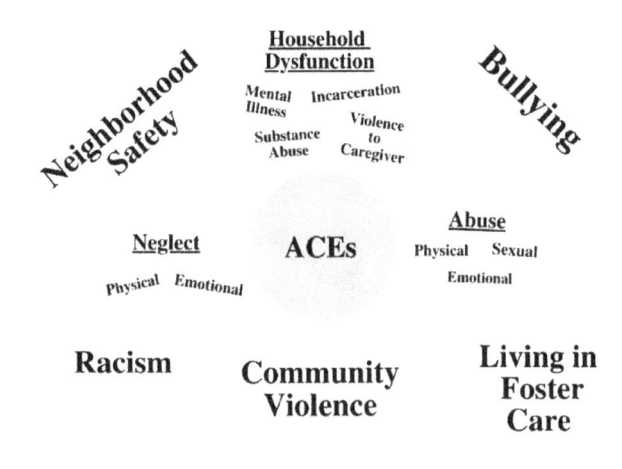

- Neighborhood Safety
- Household Dysfunction: Mental Illness, Incarceration, Substance Abuse, Violence to Caregiver
- Bullying
- Abuse: Physical, Sexual, Emotional
- Living in Foster Care
- Community Violence
- Racism
- Neglect: Physical, Emotional

Source: Cronholm, P. F., Forke, C. M., Wade, R., Bair-Merritt, M. H., Davis, M., Harkins-Schwarz, M., Pachter, L. M., & Fein, J. A. (2015). Adverse childhood experiences: Expanding the concept of adversity. American Journal of Preventive Medicine, 49(3), 354–361.

Findings from the Philadelphia Urban ACE Survey, based on a racially and socially diverse population. This study added external social factors to the ACE measures.

Not everyone who has ACEs develops severe addiction. Not everyone with severe addiction has ACEs. According to experts on psychological trauma, the 80% correlation between ACEs and addiction is more robust than random chance. What you need to know is that a relationship that strong is rare and shows the high quality of data collected in these studies.

It's clear from the charts that follow that as your ACEs go up, so do your chances of many different long-term health effects.

What's Your Score?

Prior to your 18th birthday:[20]

1. Did a parent or other adult in the household often or very often...
Swear at you, insult you, put you down, or humiliate you? or Act in a way that made you afraid that you might be physically hurt?
No___
If Yes, enter 1 __

2. Did a parent or other adult in the household often or very often...
Push, grab, slap, or throw something at you? or Ever hit you so hard that you had marks or were injured?
No___
If Yes, enter 1 __

3. Did an adult or person at least 5 years older than you ever...
Touch or fondle you or have you touch their body in a sexual way? or Attempt or actually have oral, anal, or vaginal intercourse with you?
No___

---

[20] This comes from the CDC, which allows free use of the ACE test. Here's a great resource: https://numberstory.org/explore-your-number/

If Yes, enter 1 __

4. Did you often or very often feel that ...
No one in your family loved you or thought you were important or special? or Your family didn't look out for each other, feel close to each other, or support each other?
No___If
Yes, enter 1 __

5. Did you often or very often feel that ...
You didn't have enough to eat, had to wear dirty clothes, and had no one to protect you? or Your parents were too drunk or high to take care of you or take you to the doctor if you needed it?
No___
If Yes, enter 1 ___

6. Were your parents ever separated or divorced?
No___
If Yes, enter 1 ___

7. Was your mother or stepmother:
Often or very often pushed, grabbed, slapped, or had something thrown at her? or Sometimes, often, or very often kicked, bitten, hit with a fist, or hit with something hard? or Ever repeatedly hit over at least a few minutes or threatened with a gun or knife?
No___
If Yes, enter 1 ___

8. Did you live with anyone who was a problem drinker or alcoholic, or who used street drugs?
No___
If Yes, enter 1 ___

9. Was a household member depressed or mentally ill, or did a household member attempt suicide?
No___
If Yes, enter 1 ___

10. Did a household member go to prison?
No___
If Yes, enter 1 ___

To calculate your ACE score, give yourself 1 point for each of the questions that you answered Yes: _____

Before we talk about what the ACE score means, you need to understand something. You are not your score. Here, let me put that in a Key Takeaway for you. It's important. Did I mention that? Alright, pin this up on your wall. Ready? Repeat after me:

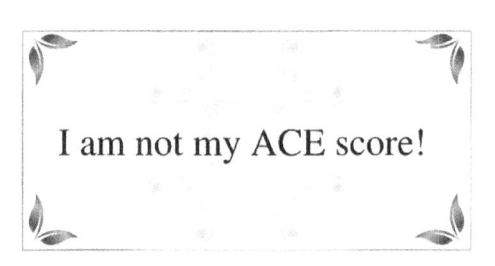

> I am not my ACE score!

My ACE score is high, or probably 9 or 10. I'm the type that can rationalize test answers, so it's one or the other. When your ACEs are high, you're probably going to wind up getting high—a lot. This was true for me.

Any way you look at it, the fact that I'm alive and can speak two coherent sentences in a row is sort of impossible. My doctor once told me that the patients she had with my history were all pushing shopping carts downtown. Then she said, "I'm not supposed to do this, but can I give you a hug?"

If I were to over-identify with my ACE score, that would make knowing about the score more of a problem than a solution. So, we don't want to use this knowledge as a weapon against ourselves. There are many aspects of self that we will get into. You have relationships with all the parts of you. As with all relationships, deep compassion is necessary. The war inside our heads can come to an end. We can make peace with our "selves."

The aspect of self that's damaged from trauma may be buried within you somewhere, unable to move. Or maybe it claws at your back door while you try to recover. There are infinite possibilities of how this stuff manifests.

In Compassionate Recovery, we can learn to accept all the parts of ourselves. Ultimately, down the road on the recovery-mastery spectrum, we can invite everybody within us—one at a time—to the table for a peaceful conversation.

Drop into Self-compassion

I know this can be challenging stuff to process. Would you join me for a Self-Compassion moment? Once you learn to do this, you'll be able to drop in when you need to. Don't worry about how long it takes. Read this, commit it to memory, then close your eyes and do the practice. If you rather, leave your eyes open half-mast, but very still.

Place your hand on your heart. Come up with your own, but here's a mantra[21] to get you started. Say it out loud, with your eyes closed. Say, "I accept all of me." Or you could sing yourself the tune but change

---

21 Here, a mantra can be any short word or phrase that you repeat out loud, quietly or silently. It's a self-soothing tool, for which a whole book could be written. Many have!

the words to something like, "All of me, accepts all of me, all my curves and imperfections...."[22]

Wow, so yeah. That was tough to feel all that stuff. It's OK to be right here, right now, and feel just this. Present to just the way it is right now. Inhale, exhale open mouth, let it all out and feel cleansed and free. This is part of the ongoing life practice of self-compassion. It's a process. You're doing great.

---

[22] Inspired by All of Me, John Stephens, Tobias Gad Lyrics © BMG Rights Management, Sony/ATV Music Publishing LLC

Notes

Chapter 3
Effects of ACEs

"A righteous student came and asked me to reflect
He judged my lifestyle was politically incorrect
I don't believe in self-important folks who preach
No Bad Religion song can make your life complete
You'll get no direction from me
You'll get no direction from me"[23]
-Bad Religion

It's vital not to over-identify with the suffering aspect of our situation. This frees up our energy to apply a compassionate solution to our problem. Now that that's settled let us look at some of the relevant results of the ACE study. We'll narrow the focus on how ACEs relate to attachment-addiction. Then we'll talk about trauma. We need to unpack how trauma and toxic stress on the brain and our nervous system can affect us for the rest of our lives. Don't worry; we also focus on solutions. While we're on the topic of the brain, we'll connect what we know about trauma's unhealthy effects on the

---
23 "No Direction," Greg Graffin, lyrics © Warner Chappell Music, Inc

brain with compassion's healing effects on the brain.

Key Findings

The following three key findings from the ACE study begin the conversation on the effects of ACEs. The participants ranged in age and were 19-60+, evenly split between males and females. However, 74.8% were white and in an affluent area. Remember, this was San Diego. Let's just start with a heavy chunk of truth from this study. An ACE score of 6 shaves 20 years off your life. Don't worry; you can get some of that back as you recover. This work is about hope.

The main findings that the researchers considered real mind-blowers were:

"1. There was a direct link between childhood trauma and adult onset of chronic disease, as well as mental illness, doing time in prison, and work issues, such as absenteeism.

2. About two-thirds of the adults in the study had experienced one or more types of adverse childhood experiences. Of those, 87 percent had experienced 2 or more types. This showed that people who had an alcoholic father, for example, were likely to have also experienced physical abuse or verbal abuse. In other words, ACEs usually didn't happen in isolation.

3. More adverse childhood experiences resulted in a higher risk of medical, mental health and social problems as an adult."[24]

If the only reason for this book were those three points, it would be enough. These things are currently addressed at the community level in some areas like Portland, Oregon, with well-funded programs. But in terms of a comprehensive guide for recovery that anyone can access, 12-Step is the most recommended because there isn't much else that anyone can go to for free and be in active recovery after treatment. Many go straight into AA, for example, with no treatment program at all. They go "cold-turkey," sweating it out on the couch alone. It's up to you, the reader if Compassionate Recovery provides a foundation for such community-based, grass-roots support groups. Traditional meetings aren't a necessary part of this guide but are encouraged.

In the private sector, individual therapies are available—for those who have the insurance. According to a San Diego psychologist with a thriving private practice that I interviewed in San Diego, most good therapists have gone to cash-only payments. Because of the limitations of the insurance industry, they often don't have much

---

24   https://acestoohigh.com/2012/10/03/the-adverse-childhood-experiences-study-the-largest-most-important-public-health-study-you-never-heard-of-began-in-an-obesi

choice. Like the hundreds of treatment providers I've spoken to about Compassionate Recovery, she loves the idea. She recognizes the need for this type of community-based support that anyone can access yet utilizes healing principles from otherwise inaccessible treatments.

The trend in residential treatment, which is primarily short-term, is to offer trauma-informed therapy, mindfulness, yoga, and other holistic therapies—only while the client is enrolled in their programs. Most of the programs are about a month-long, with some offering long-term transitional housing. The longest of those that I spoke with was about six months. So, what does the recovering addict do after that?

Post-treatment, the client is typically advised to attend 12-Step groups to maintain their recovery. But for a lifelong community-based recovery program that addresses core issues, excludes no one, and supports healing for addicts with ACES, there doesn't seem to be anything out there.

Compassionate Recovery addresses the first point directly from the beginning. It's not that people in detox for heroin should put the cart of deep-seated trauma work before the horse of getting sober, so to speak. Get off the horse. Find a mule. Go at your own pace, but don't fall off the mule. If you fall off the mule, get back on the mule. If the mule won't walk, find another mule. When your journey takes you to the place where it's time to do some work, you'll know where to start. It's important to have a big picture of the landscape, wherever we are heading on our path.

If you have an ACE score of 0, your chances of developing alcoholism over the course of adulthood are about 3%. When the score goes up to 1, your chances double to 6%. If your ACE is four or above, your chances are about 500% higher of becoming an alcoholic than if you didn't have an ACE score. Another way of saying it is that you'd be six times more likely to become an alcoholic with an ACE over four than if it were zero. The trend line shows that the rate of increase is close to exponential, but not quite the rate of IV drug use, where the impact of ACEs is truly exponential af.

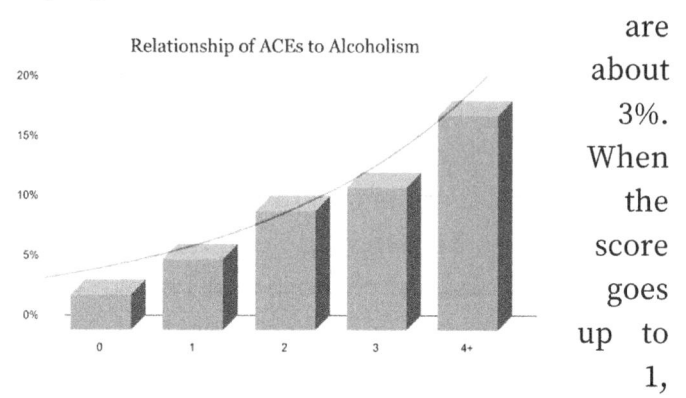

The Y Axis is the percentage, and as in the other chart, ACE scores are on the X-Axis. At ACE 0, you're about .03% likely to shoot up some dope at some point in your life. So, check out the impact of this point. This is the incontrovertible sledgehammer that clarifies why we're having this conversation. Let me know how it lands.

If your ACE score is four or higher, you're 46 times more likely to become an IV drug user than if your score is zero. This is an example of exponential growth.[25] Things get out of control faster than shit through a goose when something grows exponentially. By the time you realize you're in a mess, you look down and see that you're knee-deep in kaka. That's how it is to work with our ACEs. Don't miss this next point. If you are on the attachment-addiction spectrum somewhere, in recovery for a long time, or just thinking about it—it doesn't matter—please give yourself a pass. The struggle is real. You can't judge

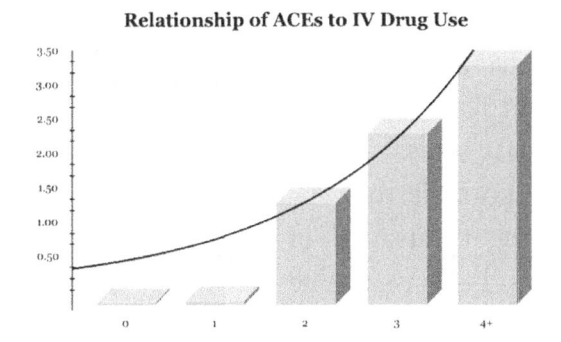

---

25 The classic example of exponential growth is the following problem. If a chessboard were to have wheat placed on each square, so that one grain is placed on the first square, two on the second, four on the third, and so on (doubling the number of grains on each subsequent square), how many grains of wheat would be on the chessboard at the finish? You'll have to guess, then Google.

yourself on how you're doing at any given point because, as we'll continue to talk about, the impact of trauma is varied and comes up in unexpected ways that you'd never think were connected to your ACEs. But they're connected to your ACEs. Know that and practice self-compassion around it. You've already started the healing process. That's what this work is about.

Our brains are plastic in that they can grow new cells and change with training. With the practices in this book, your brain can repair and rebuild in the areas that have been damaged by ACEs and long-term toxic stress. The brain can rewire itself if we learn to direct it! This is how to heal and unwind the symptoms of toxic stress.

The second point is that ACEs don't happen in isolation. Among thousands of recovering people that I've known, I can't say I've met many that *just* had an alcoholic father or *just* saw their mom get beat up. A shit show on Sunday is usually still a shit show on Tuesday. When we add societal factors, the complexity of factors influencing trauma is clearly not made up of isolated incidents but rather ongoing, pervasive stress that transcends family, school, or church.

Families who suffer from these dynamics aren't just a little bit affected. Families are systems that live in larger community systems that are part of larger social, governmental, economic, and legal systems. The causes of events that lead to trauma can't be isolated to just one member of a family, a neighborhood, or a wider community. In 2013, the

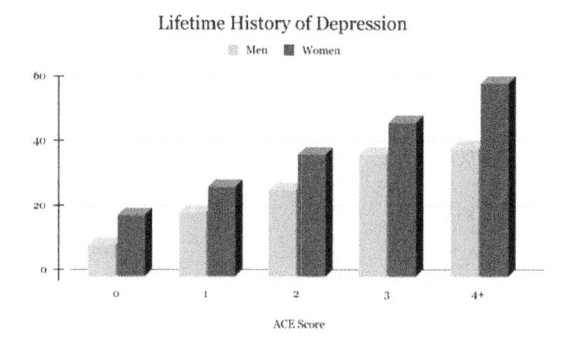

Lifetime History of Depression
Men ■ Women

[Bar chart showing increasing percentages by ACE Score from 0 to 4+]

ACE Score

Philadelphia Urban ACE study revealed the underlying social impact outside the home. Neighborhood Safety, Bullying, Racism, Community Violence and Living in Foster Care were all found in this 2012 study to be significant contributing factors that weren't considered in the first ACE study in the mid-90s.

The third finding that more adverse childhood experiences resulted in a higher risk of medical, mental health, and social problems as an adult is critical information for us as we proceed through the adult life cycle on our way to a more settled, easy place. The chances of acute effects in the later parts of life that result from ACEs are pretty much inevitable. If you're someone who has a high ACE score and is doing fine, as they say in AA, "Our hats are off to you." Remember, we can make remarkable changes in how we feel if we do the work. You can do it, and you don't have to do it alone.

Depression

If you're a woman, your chances of developing a history of depression over the course of your life are around 10% with no ACEs. With four ACEs and above, there's a four-fold increase up to a 40% chance of developing depression problems. For men, you can see that the trend is the same. As ACEs go up, so do the chances of depression. But for men, these manifestations of depression are less likely.

Suicide

As ACEs go up, so do the chances that a suicide attempt will happen at some point in your life. Does that mean everyone with an ACE of 4 or above will attempt suicide? No. As with all these findings, there is variability. The data tells us what the probability is, not a foregone conclusion. Regardless, there is a solution. Keep reading.

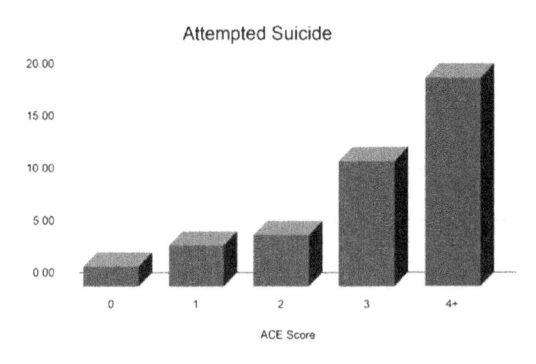

Impaired Work and Finances

A person with an ACE of 1 has about a 14% chance of serious money issues in their adult life. At four or above, someone would have almost a 25% chance of not developing good money management skills.

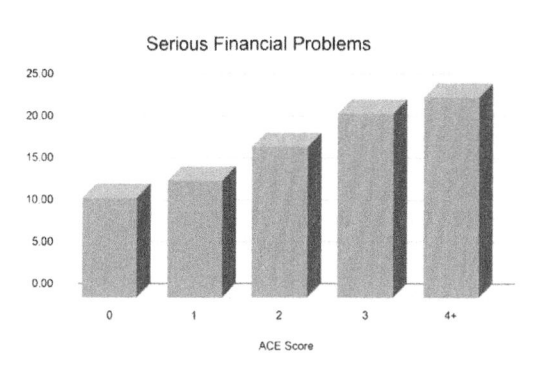

The next graph shows that in terms of employability, the picture (like all the rest), paints a salient and painfully lucid image for us. ACEs go up, and so does economic instability. Is it a guarantee? No. We can learn new skills!

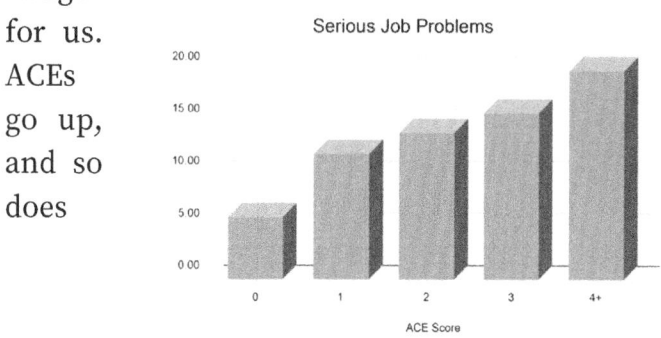

Risk of Perpetrating Domestic Violence

The X-axis is still ACEs, but we count five columns in this graph: 0,1,2,3,4,5 and above. Men are more likely to commit DV, but here's a point to consider. Did you think the chance of being a perpetrator was that high for women? Most people don't. The courts don't. And the police person does not care about this chart. If the police respond to a DV call[26] and a male is present at the complaint's location, said male goes to jail. Good luck with bail. This isn't the place to write another book on the topic, but it needs to be noted that

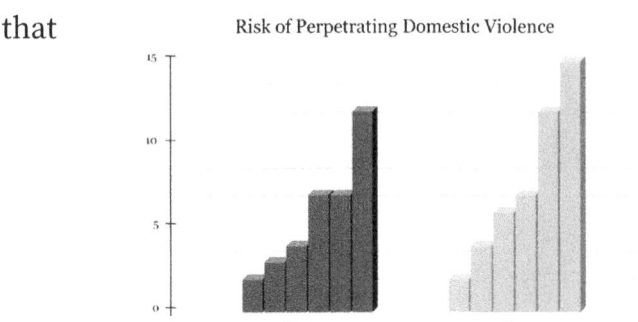

Risk of Perpetrating Domestic Violence

women are also more likely to commit Domestic Violence the higher their ACE score and that they're not far behind the bad boys in terms of bad things for the relationship.

There are many more graphs and hundreds of studies with more data than could fit many volumes.

---
26 But hey, feel free to take this book out and show the officer!

We include what is most relevant to the attachment-addiction spectrum. Please review the resources here for further research.

It's Not Your Fault

This kind of information can be disconcerting to anyone. For someone in long-term recovery, you may feel like you've done all the work yet don't understand why you still don't feel great. It may be due to some of these experiences and the resultant impairment in certain aspects of brain development. The effects often mount as we get older. The good news is that you don't' have to suffer. There's work you can do that will open the doors of relief. It's not because you didn't try hard enough or aren't committed. The fact that you have trouble functioning is not due to your lack of qualities as a person. When abuse, neglect, and other toxic stress experiences happen to us, it's not because we deserved it.

It's never, under any circumstances, ever, no matter who tells you, and regardless of what you feel about yourself, it is never your fault that you got abused. Crisis response workers know all too well that sexual assault is vastly underreported because of how difficult it is for victims of the crime to come forward due to fears of being blamed for somehow causing their assault. It's called Victim Blaming.

Victim Blaming is a harsh defense mechanism that lawyers for defendants of sexual assault crimes use to discredit the victim. It, unfortunately, thrives as part of systemic sexism and racism. We mustn't Victim Blame ourselves. That's precisely what narcissistic abusers would want. But when an assault happens, our systems can freeze the moment to exclude all but minor details, like the smell of the attacker's shampoo. They can't remember his face, just the smell, and the terror. This can be used to discredit the witness, but fortunately, there's a way to make police, the courts, and juries

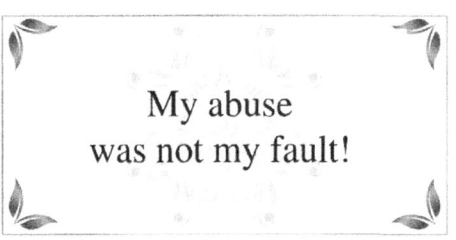

> My abuse was not my fault!

understand the trauma response at a neurological level. The response described above is normal and, to be expected, not used to harm the victim further.

Dr. Jim Hopper is an expert in this field of neuropsychology. His focus is scientific testimony in defense of victims of sexual assault trials. His brilliant way of describing the ultra-complex ways that trauma affects our brains is called The Key Brain Circuitries. This tool we'll use to demystify our experiences and give meaning to the principles and practices that Compassionate Recovery uses.

But remember, as far as science goes, we're on a need-to-know basis. Whatever you read here is a bare-bones explanation sufficient to bring the healing down to our bone marrow. If you want to know more, the weeds get very deep. If you really want to gain expertise, there are quite a few opportunities for research in the field of trauma research.

I think you'll agree that the mention of this significant point warrants a memorable graphic symbol to burn the idea onto our mental EPROMs.[27] So let's burn this message right in there where the circuits connect.

ACEs can create a compounded, developmental trauma that pushes us along our various spectrums and dimensions, ready or not. If one part of the brain relies on another part of the brain, but that other part has some problems due to trauma in childhood, the difficulties will compound or pile up on each other over time. For example, social development issues influence learning problems. If we're not emotionally ready to advance a grade, our performance may decline academically because ACEs affect whole brain development. What looks like learning disabilities in grammar school may become behavior problems in high school, if not

---

27 Erasable, programmable, Read Only Mental Memory, based on the idea of the EPROM, in full erasable programmable read-only memory, form of computer memory that does not lose its content when the power supply is cut off and that can be erased and reused. EPROMs can be upgraded with a later version of a program. EPROMs are erased with ultraviolet light. The capabilities of EPROMs were later extended with EEPROM (electrically erasable programmable read-only memory. EEPROM. https://www.britannica.com/technology/EPROM Think of the tools in this book as an EEPROM – extend those capabilities baby!

sooner. We don't have to look very far to see examples of this everywhere, in and out of our own families.

High ACEs are like building a skyscraper with no wiring or structural support on some floors. Some stairwells are missing. Other routes always seem to be blocked. It's hard to get to the top floor if each level isn't constructed according to plan, whether that top floor is a happy relationship with oneself or the ability to be attachment-addiction free.

Here's the deal. Old school recovery approaches had no idea what to do with this reality. High ACEs impacted our chances of falling into the deeper end of the attachment-addiction spectrum and inhibited our ability to move out of white-knuckle sobriety into long-term spiritual contentment. But with the tools we had, many survived. As we've discussed, many do not.

We were, after all, a bunch of drunks in church basements filled with cigarette smoke. There were very few among us who didn't have ACEs. We had no language for it and no preview of the long-term effects. For example, people in long-term sobriety often suffer from debilitating depression. Some commit suicide—we can all name someone we know who's been affected by this. I want you to let this one sink in. Keep this point in mind. Don't ever forget it.

Traumatic childhood events can cause molecular changes in your brain chemistry. People in long-term recovery haven't had this awareness or a support system to educate and sustain recovery through this widespread problem of long-term effects. No matter how hard we've worked in our conventional recovery approaches, these deep issues have been elusive to our understanding until now.

We can now assemble a framework to understand the impact of our childhood experiences on the different aspects of ourselves and the connection to our place(s) on an attachment-addiction spectrum. We kept telling each other to keep coming back and not drink in between meetings.

It wasn't until the early 90s that the technology emerged to help scientists see the brain in ways that broke loose knowledge of brain functioning. This technology has allowed researchers to dig deep into our brains to figure out the direct links between ACES and our experiences as addicts. This should be very clear by the time you finish this book. In fact, you'll have useful knowledge to help others.

Everything contained here is meant to be integrated with practice. If you scan the book and say, "Yeah, it's OK. I didn't do the practices, but it was interesting, " I've unfortunately failed you. The point should be clear; this material isn't worth a whole hell of a lot if it's just words on paper.[28] We will need to apply the medicine directly to our core

---

28 Unless you live in Texas during a winter blackout. If something like that happens—please—feel free to burn this book to stay warm.

wounds to get the healing results. All of this connects to brain research on compassion and mindfulness practices pertaining to the condition we find ourselves in.

We can see that many problems occur—including a propensity to get high—if we have high ACEs. But what exactly happens to us when we have these experiences? How do these events shape our ability to function physically, mentally, emotionally, and spiritually? There's a lot to learn about the brain, but the information we have now is substantially, enormously, and incredibly higher quality and more voluminous than ever before in the history of addiction. In twenty years, we'll know more. But this picture is clear. We're developing this story. Now we see the ACE story. We have an idea of our own ACEs if we have any. In our knowledge base (KB) that we're developing, we know that if we have ACEs, it affects our brains in unhealthy ways that have a lifelong impact. We have an understanding now of some of the core causes of attachment-addiction. Of course, there are genetic factors and so forth. We really can't do anything about that here. But we can do some healing if you're willing to walk through the pain because you have to feel the pain to heal the pain. We've lived with it all of our lives so that we can walk through this.

To get better, we need precise knowledge. How granular to get on this stuff is a decision you'll have to make. After combing through hundreds of research papers, books, and clinicians and researchers, this is the clear, essential information that I think is important to the journey. I'm not a brain scientist, and this is a layman's synopsis of specialized technical material.

You might feel like you need a degree in neuroscience to understand what's going on in your brain, but you don't. Here we're on a need-to-know basis. We need to know enough to apply the information to our healing. Compassionate Recovery is designed to be accessible and something anyone can work with yet considers the latest brain research. The critical part of understanding the Key Brain Circuitries is developing a Compassionate Recovery Roadmap of specific meditations and other practices. Brain science shows that these practices are like a medicinal salve on our raw, festering wounds. This will be the ongoing life application of all the information we're gathering here.

Live and learn. Learn and heal. Heal and help others.

Compassion practice is dose-related. It works on a logarithmic dose-response curve, like how the efficacy of pharmaceuticals is measured. The ideal effectiveness is that the more doses of the medicine you take, the higher the desired result, i.e., we feel better. Simply put, the more we apply *consistent* practice, the more we grow. Like a spiral builds on itself, the more we grow, the faster we grow.

Practice changes things.

The bottom lines:
- Your brain can heal using the practices and principles in this book.
- Principles are laws or rules that can be counted on, like gravity.
- Practices are applications of these principles.

Here, the work will heal your brain, heart, mind, and soul. It's hard af, not going to lie. But you can do it. You're a badass. Come on now, let's rock this! OK, so maybe you're not feeling it quite yet. This is complex material to cover. Let's take the wisdom from our earlier epigraph and turn it into a self-healing, narrative changing, nervous system enhancing, and super cool practice.

Drop into Self-compassion

Find a calm space, if possible, in a calm place. Think about the smaller person that you were during adverse childhood experiences. If you don't have any ACEs, imagine what you might have felt like if you experienced those things at that time in your life. Imagine yourself at that age, in a room in a chair. Enter that space and ask if you can sit for a moment. Look yourself in the eye or however you feel you can connect and say, hey, I know you want and need to hear some things, so I'm going to say these things to you, and I mean them, OK? Then say this slowly. Make meaning.

Put your hand on your heart. Say the words
I believe in you.
You have worth.
You can do hard things.
You are loved (or I love you).

Notes

Chapter 4
ACEs and Recovery

"She generally gave herself very good advice, (though she very seldom followed it)"
– Alice's Adventures in Wonderland

This book is for everyone in any stage of attachment to addiction. It's also for those already in recovery looking for a spark and have the courage to take a step forward. Before we get into the details of trauma and the brain, let's put ACEs and attachment-addiction in the perspective of long-term recovery. It makes sense to see the long view as we chart our roadmap of recovery. It doesn't mean we have to do the deeper work right away. But at least it won't knock you upside the head in your eighth year sober. You'll be prepared if you lay the foundation in this book.

For the sake of clarity, I've chosen to illustrate the effects of ACEs in the long term because it's closest to my own experience. We will discuss the recovery-mastery spectrum in Part III.

We will cover The Funnel, The Spiral, Triggers, and Backdraft. Each section has a suggested practice to internalize, connect and *make meaning*[29] of the work. Before we dig in too deeply, I want to encourage you to create or revisit your Circle of Safety network. Long-term research on addiction shows that social support is critical to success in recovery.[30]

However, when embarking on this path, we get into serious topics quickly. It's a good idea to establish support for this path, even if you already have recovery support.

Circle of Safety

The circle of safety is a group of people that you choose. With each individually, you make an honest agreement for ongoing or temporary support with some aspect of your recovery process. If you have one person, you trust with everything, that's fine.

---

29 Quoted in Park, C. L. (2010). Making sense of the meaning literature: An integrative review of meaning making and its effects on adjustment to stressful life events. Psychological Bulletin, 136(2), 257–301. https://doi.org/10.1037/a0018301

"From "Baumeister (1991) proposed a reasonable definition of meaning as a "mental representation of possible relationships among things, events, and relationships. Thus, meaning connects things" (p. 15). Although difficult to define, the notion of meaning as central to human life is a popular one. Meaning appears particularly important in confronting highly stressful life experiences, and much recent research has focused on meaning making (i.e., the restoration of meaning in the context of highly stressful situations)." So make your work meaningful by doing the practices!

30 Moos, R., & Timko, C. (2008). Outcome research on twelve-step and other self-help programs. In M. Galanter, & H. O. Kleber (Eds.), Textbook of substance abuse treatment (4th ed. pp. 511-521). Washington, DC: American Psychiatric Press.

But I'm asking you to expand your safety net. Don't get a second opinion. Get five or six. In your circle, you will need people in recovery, and you also need people who are not in recovery. A family member or spouse is fine for part of your support, but it is not healthy, nor does it work out to expect one person to handle our whole load. It's not fair to them, and it doesn't work. Spread your needs out among the four dimensions.

One member can be a workout buddy who is informed about recovery and the importance of maintaining good physical condition. Another would be more of an emotional support person. They can agree to be there to simply listen or offer advice—whatever the two of you work out.

The relationship with each member is set up intentionally and upfront to be mutually beneficial. You don't get to drain half a dozen people energetically and offer nothing in return. That is not how it works. In fact, it's more the reverse. Try to offer more than you ask for.

To approach a new member of your circle, find a way to offer service to them. When you request to be in your circle, tell them that this is not a one-way relationship. You must give back in a mutually agreed-upon exchange of energy. Walk their dog. Wash their truck. Babysit or do some shopping. There is always a way to give back. This type of compassionate exchange is essential because addicts and people with high ACEs can suck the life out of people close to them. You know it as well as I do. That's why this approach has served me for over thirty years.

Ask the person if they would be willing to spend fifteen minutes with you or exchange some emails/texts to discuss this. Write down why you chose them and tell them about it when you meet. Explain briefly what you're working on, how it helps your recovery, and why you'd love it if they'd be on your trusted team. If you need help writing this up in advance, find a buddy and work on it together!

Find a mental friend once you have the physical and emotional support set up. A mental friend can be anyone you can do something with that you both enjoy, that serves them and your recovery, and most importantly, the activity must make you smarter. Choose a trip to the bookstore or museum, watch an art film, or work on a game or puzzle. The idea is to connect on the thinking level with a support person. This person can be there to listen to your best ideas, point out flaws in your logic, or support you where you feel weak. Recovery happens in four dimensions of humanity. Your job is to serve and nurture each.

The fourth dimension, spirituality, is open to any being that makes you feel something spiritual. I can't define that for you. It could be a teacher, alive or dead. It might be a lover, your garden, or your dog[31].

---

[31] Tip: if your dog chose you to be your spiritual support, I've found that chicken jerky treats work really well as an energy exchange.

This is your personal spiritual support being. Find and nurture your spiritual feeling with someone that you can connect with. It's incredible and life-changing, so be sure to set it up!

What about meetings as support? We're going to address the community in a later section. What we need to know at the moment is that Compassionate Recovery is meant to be used in diverse ways. It's not just another book to base a meeting on.

First, it's a personal guide to full spectrum recovery. You don't have to go out and find a whole new community. Take this book with you to your current treatment, 12-Step program, or other support groups. Seek out like minds interested in talking about some of this work. Most of the key takeaways are simple ideas that you can use to strike up a conversation with someone at a meeting, the circle of safety, for example.

Most 12-Step formats recommend one person to serve as a sponsor, who will guide you through the steps in the order they are written, based on their own experience. The circle of safety takes a wider, safer approach than putting all your trust eggs in one other addict's basket. If you have people that deserve your trust, that's wonderful. But for many of us, trust is easily broken, and you're left shaken and traumatized from yet another betrayal. It isn't necessary to take these risks if you have high ACEs. You can build your own network, provided you're truthful with every person. You build integrity in relationships by never lying, scamming, or gaming anyone. Over time the trust builds, and deep, lifelong relationships form. Besides, when you think about it, it isn't even possible to have one person serve all of your recovery needs. How do we approach this in our current meetings?

Make connections with people who would like to work with you on the side from your regular program or as an enhancement to it. Not everyone will be into it, but you don't need to leave your current program to build this team. Find a couple of sober buddies and have informal meetups in person or online. Start where you can, but you must start. Remember, consistency is key. Repeat good behaviors. Develop new habits. Share these with others. Help others do this work.

Second, Compassionate Recovery meeting formats are available later in the book. Meetings, however, are not the main focus of this book. Rather than depend on one type of group, it's more important to learn to connect with wider humanity in meaningful ways to support our recovery. This is about connection and meaning. Meaningful connection is what saves us. Compassion is the key to meaningful connection. When someone wants to connect with you, it's for a reason. Try to be open and explore with someone you may not usually talk to. Make connections. Find the ones that will work for you for a close circle of safety that will get you through hard times and tough decisions. Don't try to find people to justify your bullshit, though. It won't be a recovery action. We want to take new actions for new results.

Recovery Practice: Circle of Safety List

List out 3-5 people you would like to include in your circle of safety. Start a preliminary list of the qualities you want in your trusted people. When considering these characteristics, choose people who have qualities that you admire and desire. Below is a simple exercise to help you get started.

Fill in the chart with the qualities you want in a member of your safety circle in the top row, then fill in the blanks. This can be a process that changes over time. For now, make a start.

Good listener	Supports LGBTQ	High integrity	Compassionate
Joanne	Juan	Darnell	Dannie
Andrea	Joanne	Joanne	Luke
Luke	Luke	Andrea	Joanne

Draft a note to these people explaining why you find them to be valuable to you. Ask if they'd like to be a part of your trusted circle. Do this first with people you know, such as family members or your counselor. Email or text them your note and let them know that you value them and what you value them for and what you would need from them. Here's an example, but please craft your own:

"Luke, as you may know, I value you as a friend. For my recovery program, I'm creating a Circle of Safety. I value your support of women and people of color and that you're an honest and compassionate person. Would you consider being in my inner circle to help me feel empowered in my recovery? That means that I'd ask for your advice and would agree to follow it, even if it's against what I'm feeling at the moment. I'll put my trust in you. You know how I am when it comes to relationships! I understand if it's too much, and I still value you as a friend."

Have fun with your circle of safety. The whole point is to support you in your journey in a reciprocal way. Make sure to connect with your members consistently and truthfully. It will help keep out from slipping into the funnel.

The Funnel

As we've seen, ACEs can dramatically increase our chances of getting on the attachment-addiction spectrum. But it can also decrease our ability to stay in recovery long-term. Addiction doesn't happen in a straight line. Neither does recovery. When we understand that growth happens in a spiral, we may be able to avoid falling into The Funnel.

In the original presentation of The Funnel[32], I framed it as something that happens after nearly a decade of sobriety. But with this new information, it's clear that this cycle can explain what happens with those chronic relapsers, those men and women unable to get any recovery at all. It would make sense that those in long-term recovery would have dealt with this kind of thing, and to a degree, many have.

But here's the twist.

ACEs are about the long-term impact on adult humans over the life cycle. In later years, which, as we have seen, can be decades shorter due to ACEs, we do tend to lose some of our defenses. The older we get, the more of an imprint our ACEs can have.

Ted was 12 years sober in AA down in Long Beach in the 90s. He was a decent guy, always helping others in the program. I'd see Ted every night at the meeting, making coffee for the group. One night I realized I hadn't seen Ted in a while, so I asked

---

[32] The 12-Step Buddhist (2009, 2018 Atria\Beyond Words)

around. Since this was the first time I'd known someone in recovery experienced this, I was hardcore shocked to find out that Ted had killed himself. Nobody knew why. He was an active member of the fellowship. Worked his steps and everything. There wasn't a framework around trauma and addiction to give us an understanding at that time.

We can't know why Ted took his life. But we know he was an alcoholic and that ACEs are related to alcoholism and don't happen alone. In that case, it's not a bad guess that Ted ran into severe mental and emotional issues even in the absence of their object of attachment-addiction.

Scott and Amy, another couple that I knew, got clean together in the early 2000s. They spent about 19 years doing life sober and being at ease. Just before he was ready to retire, Scott became distant. He eventually relapsed into hard-core addiction and overdosed. When Amy, understandably devastated, wrote about it on her social media, she said that there was no other man for her after Scott. He was her soulmate right till the end, even though they hadn't even been together for several years. The work here can spare some of us from these fates.

ACEs can drop us into The Funnel even when working hard on recovery. That's why we need to know about them and address the trauma from the beginning, even if it takes a while to heal. The phenomenon of relapse, life collapse, and suicide has never really been dealt with in the recovery rooms that I've seen. People I've met on the road of recovery tend to dismiss these things as a lack of willingness or somehow falling out of the rigorous routine of meetings and service seven days a week that keep most recovering addicts glued to their groups for fear of falling off the wagon. Yet, for some, regardless of our efforts and the cries of those around us, we fall off the wagon anyways, right into The Funnel.

Most people don't fall into The Funnel. Some people are just stable by nature after they stop their addictions. Others don't dig too deep into childhood issues once they do the 12 Steps because they're satisfied where they are.

When we fall off the track, it's devastating. Some fall into depression, despair, lack of joy, or general dissatisfaction despite all our effort and progress. It can make us question why we got sober in the first place. The typical advice typically doesn't make us feel better when it's like this. It's difficult for traditional talk therapy to affect the root causes substantially. We may seek out more charged-up activities like making more money, having more sex, or gambling with higher-than-normal risks.

But if we wake up in The Funnel one morning, maybe next to a dumpster in Tijuana with a handcuff on one wrist, sans pants. If something that crazy happens to us, does it mean that we're hopeless and have no chance to recover?

No, it doesn't mean that.

It just feels like that.

We can avoid The Funnel or learn the skills to get ourselves up out of it. But first, we must know that it's a set of roadblocks on the path for many people. Even if we don't have to deal with this ourselves, it is

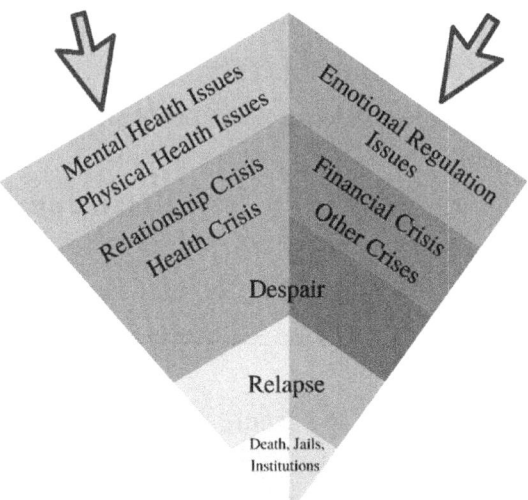

Funnel diagram showing tiers: Mental Health Issues, Physical Health Issues, Relationship Crisis, Health Crisis, Emotional Regulation Issues, Financial Crisis, Other Crises → Despair → Relapse → Death, Jails, Institutions

vital to be aware of it in our efforts to support others.

The Funnel isn't necessarily a guaranteed straight drop to the end. We can cycle through different parts of it many times. We dip in and out of life struggles. The first tier or danger zone is when we experience the effects of our ACEs that set us up for addiction and subsequent challenges in recovery. The second tier could be any crisis, stressful event, or combination that happens as a result. When our stress tolerance breaks down, we can sink into depression or have a manic phase, sending us up to or into the Relapse Funnel, cycling through The

Funnel until we change the cycle, or the cycle kills us—whichever comes first.

The stress on an already challenged brain can tip us over the edge of The Funnel if we aren't aware of the big picture and have a detailed plan to stay on the balance beam of recovery. We'll see parts of ourselves from different points of view as we move through life. The physical body is an easy example. Time affects everyone in ultimately the same way.

Integration Practice: Funnel Factors

If you're brand new to recovery, file this practice for down the road. When clarity is needed, this can be an ongoing practice skill that you use as a reality checkpoint. Look at the image of The Funnel.

Considering what we've learned so far, assess what mental, physical, or emotional factors can suck you down the funnel. Write out some real or hypothetical scenarios. Share them with friends in recovery. Ask what their funnel factors are.

One way to avoid falling into The Funnel starts with knowing where the funnel factors are so that you can plan on your Roadmap of Recovery.

The Spiral

Most of us can relate to spiraling emotionally to one degree or another. But spirals aren't always downward. The poet Yeats thought that spirals could go forward and backward like two cones facing each other[33]. Spirals can be seen as the structures of the tiniest DNA to the farthest galaxies[34]. The salient characteristic of the spiral is that it goes forward and backward at the same time. We return to a starting point on any number of aspects, features, or qualities, but growth or decay has occurred, just like a Saturn Return.

We can experience and part of us, for example, our Angry Self, as a sort of Saturn Return, where after thirty years or so, the planet Saturn returns to the same position in the sky as it was the day of your birth. That point is the same. But you've changed. It's not always easy to see growth because sometimes it happens on a different timeline than we may expect.

Think of the little Saturn as any aspect of yourself on any four dimensions; physical, mental, emotional, or spiritual. Each successive orbit is structurally dependent on the previous orbit. That means we go along in patterns. The way that pattern is structured affects our next phase around the cycle. On a cycle, we might be in any stage with an object[35]

---

33 The Second Coming by William Butler Yeats, n.d.

34 Pruska Oldenhof, Izabella, and Robert K. Logan. 2017. "The Spiral Structure of Marshall McLuhan's Thinking" Philosophies 2, no. 2: 9. https://doi.org/10.3390/philosophies2020009

35 The object is the thing we may find sticky, problematic or totally addictive. If you want take it to another level, consider that the separateness of me (subject) and you or any other

of attachment, pre-addiction, addiction, or severe addiction. The spiral can be a template for early-middle-late-stage recovery and more of a life mastery or spiritual wholeness.

Aspects of self are any parts or characteristics, including how we respond to ACEs later in life. It may look like we're going backward, but if we keep at our program, we'll find that we come out at a higher level. Our coping ability, success in sobriety, and financial or relationship experiences can be seen in this light over time in recovery.

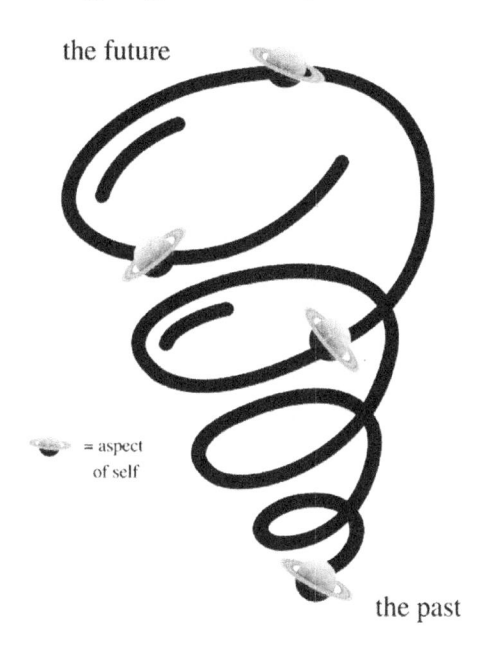

the future

= aspect of self

the past

Our relationship to traumatic events and memories can also be understood in the context of the spiral. For example, if our Saturn was a memory

---

phenomena that I consider not me, (object) is a dualistic relationship. It's a subject-object relationship between me—a little spec—and the whole rest of the infinite universe that is the problem, according to teachings on non-duality. If we can get into that kind of framework, compassion arises spontaneously.

of an event when we were three years old, we will see, feel, and have health issues from that event which have different qualities and will be from different perspectives throughout time. The event didn't change. But we did, as did our perception of that event over a period.

What's your Saturn? Recall an impactful event that you keep returning to, volitionally or spontaneously. How has it looked at different stages of your maturity? Do you feel the impact has lessened, or is it stronger now?

Our progress in dealing with traumatic experiences can feel up and down. The good news is that we can affect our current understanding of the past, but that still affects us.

Try a little practice to get a sense of your shift in awareness of a part of your body.

Drop into Spiral Memory

You may record this one or have a friend read it to you. Think of how your hands looked and felt when you first learned to ride a bike or skateboard, skip rope, or shoot a basket. Close your eyes and try to recall that moment. Remember the feelings and sensations around you then. How did you see yourself? What did you look like to you?

Open your eyes.

Look at your hands again. How are they the same as back then? Leave your hands very still for a moment. Close your eyes again and try to notice your hands. If you don't move, how do you know they're there? What is it about your hands that hasn't changed since the day you just recalled? Your hand is your hand on every point in the spiral of time and experience, growth, and decay. It may be a little mind-bending to meditate on this, but it will shift your perspective.

You can do this kind of practice with any memory. Try it with another one, the experience of safety. How is your sense of safety right now? How was it when you were seven? Use any point in your life to just go back and forth. Remember how it looked in one period of your life, but then recall the same thing from another time or another angle in your life. Shift awareness from a point in the past to the present. Then another point in the past. Shift back to the present. Try this with your general experience of specific emotions. Do the meditations for anger, sadness, hope, and joy. Travel through the spiral with your experiences to get a different perspective. This skill helps with trauma work.

The way we experience frustration, happiness, fear, and love is based on the accumulation of our past experiences. The more intense experiences are stored somehow in our bodies and conscious or unconscious memory.

When we meet difficulties, we can choose how we want to be, even if we've never felt empowered before. We can cultivate and nurture it, feel it, own it, and work from this core strength deep that we built in the center of our belly. Over time, we create a fulfilling, embodied experience with training and practice. Eventually, we can have more days where we can awaken to calm and total relief instead of waking up in shock and disbelief.

Triggers

When we think of a trigger on a gun, it usually must be pulled to cause an explosion. Not so with our triggers. They fire up parts of the brain circuitries related to the original trauma. Our inner stress response triggers trauma response switches on for known or unknown reasons. They can be unknown because ongoing trauma endured over time, rather than an isolated incident, causes our memories to get scrambled. There's no way to keep a correct temporal sequence of events beneath the surface of consciousness. Our bodies have billions of nerves that process sensory information every moment of every day. Most of it is beneath our conscious awareness.

Researchers tell us that traumatic memories get frozen deep in our brains and bodies. This can be due to a traumatic event, series of events, or long-term timeline with a mental, emotional tone of being unsafe. The sequence of traumatic experiences tends to be out of order from the original occurrence. Are we supposed to untangle all of that in talk therapy?

You can't always put these feelings to words. Think of how difficult it is in a dream to make sense of something that you try to read or if you try to tell time on a clock. You may get a creepy feeling that doesn't make sense as to why it's happening. Yet our conscious minds constantly struggle to frame a reason—not the real reason—for the feelings. We may, for example, blame ourselves. If someone asks us how we feel, and we answer that we happen to be depressed[36], the response is, "Why do you feel that way?" If we're experiencing an ACE response, it may not be possible to give an accurate answer. We might

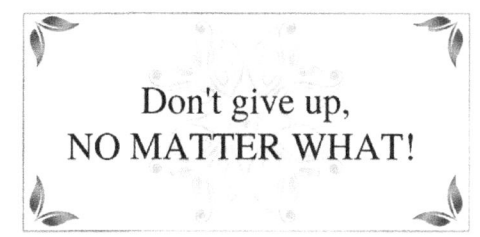

> Don't give up,
> NO MATTER WHAT!

---

[36] The same applies to other feelings such as shame, panic or rage that we can experience when triggered.

have a story about it or draw a blank when looking for answers. Don't be discouraged if this is something you identify with. There are healing tools that allow us to connect and embody our experience of life rather than frantically pursue ways to disconnect. We get down to the core of it with the practices outlined here. There are a lot of solutions to be had if we're interested in healing.

Because of this, we can experience conscious or unconscious triggers in as little as 1/8 second that switch on a trauma response—from the past—might make little or no sense because there's nothing in front of us causing that kind of feeling. Yet we feel it. It might be a love song, the sweet smell of summer, a flash of sunlight off the water, or the feeling of fabric on the back of our neck that can overwhelm our brain in what's called an Allostatic Overload[37]. This can result in a feeling based on a sensory flashback in time to what we experienced at a moment or extended period of trauma.

Kori was in recovery from heroin for six years before realizing they became nauseous and sweaty in any room with a white tile floor. After several years of somatic psychotherapy and mindfulness practice, the reason became clearer. When Kori was five to seven, their father sexually assaulted them regularly. The regular assaults often happened on the white tile floor in the laundry room of their small

---

[37] See Chapter 5

suburban home, with the whir of the Whirlpool humming somewhere far, far away.

White tile is the trigger. Triggers can bring on anything from minor anxiety to a catastrophic meltdown. They can happen unconsciously in one eight of a second. When someone asks you, "Why are you upset?" but can't answer, you possibly got triggered somehow. Maybe you beat yourself up for these kinds of reactions that defy your understanding. An alternative is to rewrite the narrative. Something like,

This feels like it's happening now.

It's not at all like that.

Say it. Know it.

And walk yourself right out of that shit.

When we do the work, we find the answers. We'll talk more about triggers soon and how to heal your wounds at the root level. Healing is painful but worth it.

If all we had to look forward to was more suffering, we'd have nothing to talk about. At ten years sober in the 90s, I fought the Funnel, and the Funnel won. I eventually crawled back up by the skin of my teeth. I got my feet on the ground, as they say. One foot in front of the other. It took time and effort to heal. But life got extremely good as a result of the work and not giving up. Do not give up. No matter what. Say it with me, out loud, with strength and conviction. Use it now or save it for a rainy day.

This mantra is like Active Shooter Training for inner self-defense. Make lists of these and use them.

I am grounded on my path, no matter what comes up.

I will never even consider giving up.

As you go on in your recovery, use the space below to add your mantras. Don't worry if they're not original. That will come. Remember, if you repeat something you hear three times, it's yours forever!

Integration Practice: Safety First

Let's put a safety on that trigger. Put your hand on your heart or another part of the body that feels tension. Say, "This is a stress response from the past. It's hard. I'm here now. I feel my hands. I feel my feet. I'm in the present moment. I'm on stable ground." Breathe with it, slow and deep as possible. Take your time. Allow yourself to relax completely. Be aware *without effort* to contain or escape this moment. It's time to release it, which means to feel it and let it go. Say this, "This is from when I was in distress. I'm safe now. It's OK to feel this right now and let it go." Stay present with your body. Notice your heartbeat. Be right there—for you. Say this, "I am safe. I am safe."

I realize that there are people in situations and institutions where it's not easy to feel safe. Put your hand on your heart and coach yourself, "This is hard. I can do hard things." Progress happens when we start right where we are, wherever we find ourselves. If we practice finding our center wherever we find ourselves, we'll be able to find our center anywhere, any time. No one will be able to move you.

"I am centered. No one can move me off my center."

Remember, practice is dose-related. Return to this on a consistent basis to yield results. What are the results? You train your brain to feel better. More relaxed. Safe.

Backdraft

Because we're addressing the trauma stored in the body, use some caution. When we get still, feelings are free to come to the surface. Depending on where you are in your life and your recovery, some practices may present more challenges. You may get what self-compassion researchers Kristin Neff and Christopher Germer

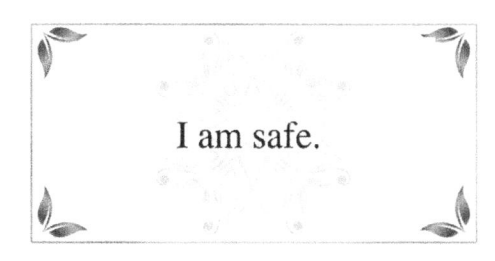

> I am safe.

call *backdraft*[38]. As a sort of participant-observer for this book and my own personal work, I took their Mindful Self-compassion (MSC) course twice for a total of 18 weeks, plus ongoing follow-up support.

The first course was the year before COVID on Zoom, with a trainer in the Netherlands. When I tried to follow her simple instructions, I felt like I was at minus zero on the self-compassion spectrum. The meditation was to simply feel warmth for myself. I was shocked that I couldn't find a thread to pull to get started.

Do you remember that wall of ice in Game of Thrones? It might have melted faster than I was going to "get" this practice. My brain didn't have the circuitry, or rather it had it, but it evaded me how to fire up the self-compassion mechanism within myself. It wasn't until nearly a year later, midway through a second 10-week MSC course, that I was able to melt the ice by retraining my mind. The breakthrough allowed me to bring healing self-compassion to myself. But it was nearly impossible without specific, guided work that took trauma into account.

Why was it such a hurdle?

As you will hear on the news around major fires, firefighters advise never to open the door to a burning room. Once new oxygen begins to feed a

---

[38] Germer, Christopher K.; Neff, Kristin D. (2013). Self-Compassion in Clinical Practice. Journal of Clinical Psychology, 69(8), 856–867. doi:10.1002/jclp.22021

contained fire, such as behind a door at the end of a hallway, the fire (of your buried wounds) can explode down the hall (your mental/emotional state) when the door (of self-inquiry) is opened, frying everything in its path (don't worry it only feels that way). That's backdraft.

Backdraft is normal when we do difficult personal work. As someone who's done extensive personal work over a lifetime, I can share that resistance to self-love isn't the only way it can show up. We didn't call it backdraft in AA and weren't trying to refine an evidence-based research principle. But we had a warning for newcomers who dove into the personal inventory process of AA's 12 Steps. This self-inquiry that is to be shared with another human being—leaving nothing out causes a lot of intensely emotional, physical, and mental responses that might result from triggers from doing the work outside a caring and trauma-educated context. Compassionate Recovery, the idea, is about creating this proper context for healing right from the beginning. Because many people, in fact, relapse after taking that step without ever completing all twelve. I would go out on a ledge and state that ACEs have a lot to do with that reaction that I've seen in my story and thousands of others in recovery rooms since 1984. With the understanding outlined here, I feel that we can compassionately clear out much of this blockage to healing.

To all of our benefit, these scientists have validated what Buddhists consider basic knowledge. Namely, that compassion is good for you, which current brain research supports. However, my Tibetan Buddhist teachers have said that it would be culturally odd for them to think of directing compassion at oneself. The idea is more about letting go of the self-cherishing ego and focusing on others. But psychologically, and especially for ACE survivors, self-compassion is the next level. Without self-compassion, we can't rock the compassion for others.

Self-compassion, then as an evidence-based, well-researched topic in psychology, is, in my opinion, an advancement in the application of some original Buddhist ideas. That, however, is not what's most important. The essential principle at hand is the main point and how to integrate it into our heart and soul by making meaning around it.

The principle we're dealing with here is unavoidable. There's no way around backdraft. You've got to feel the pain to heal the pain. It takes courage, which you already have for sure. You're not reading this by accident. How much, if any, backdraft you'll experience is hard to say. It can be a spark or a blast of emotion, positive or negative, like joy or fear. The amazing news is that the practices of compassion heal us. Here, you're invited to integrate them into your Roadmap of Compassionate Recovery, which includes known healing approaches' major principles. This is an essential part of the work.

Another vital element is social support. Line up your people. Let them know what you're embarking on. Remember, this path can't be completed in a 28-day treatment program, let alone a weekend workshop. This is a long-haul approach. That's why you're seeing the whole picture, warts and all, from the start. Sometimes it'll be uncomfortable. Don't panic. Backdraft signifies that you're getting closer to where healing is most needed. And you know that means your badassness will burst forth, and then who knows what? Are there limits? NO LIMITS. Come on now. Let's drop into the limitless present.

Drop into Being Just This Moment

The practice of compassion begins with the ability to slow down enough to be fully present to just one thing, like your body's temperature around your heart space. We eventually bring the skill of dropping into all our experiences on all dimensions, bitter or sweet. We need to slow things down and refine our noticer to be fully present. What's a noticer? It's whoever is noticing the experience without being caught up in it.

Before you begin this exercise, think about a situation that has been difficult for you to accept in the past. Let's not go to difficulty level 10 at this point. Maybe level 2 or 3. Using a journal, if possible, for ongoing work. Write down a few sentences about that person, place, or time. Then find a space where you can do a little meditation for a few minutes. Sit in a comfortable position. Let your eyes be still, half-closed. Straight back. Take a couple of deep breaths, inhale fully and let it out slowly each time.

Spend a few minutes mentally scanning your body. Wherever your awareness takes you, your body is right. Notice the sensations. If that's not too much, continue. If it's too much, practice for as long as it takes to move on to the next level. If that takes a while, that's OK. Permit yourself to grow when you grow—no need to push.

Read your journal entry about that difficult situation. Now close your eyes and imagine how you felt at the time and how you feel right now thinking about it. Breathe in slowly, breathe out slowly. Notice the body sensations. Open your eyes and let your energy settle for a moment. Where do you feel the sensation? Put your hand there if you can. Let yourself be just as you are in this moment. Don't try to change anything or fix it or analyze it. Just practice being there for a moment, as it is. As you are. If you like, you can say this three times to yourself or with a group:

Being just this moment is compassion's way.

That's one way to practice the practice of acceptance—little by little. The skill grows with experience. Some days more, others less. However it is, we can practice with it.

Notes

Part II

Trauma, Addiction, and the Brain: What We Need to Know

> "Traumatic stress isn't simply a negative emotional experience. It's an incomplete, survival-based response" David A. Treleaven. "Trauma-Sensitive Mindfulness."

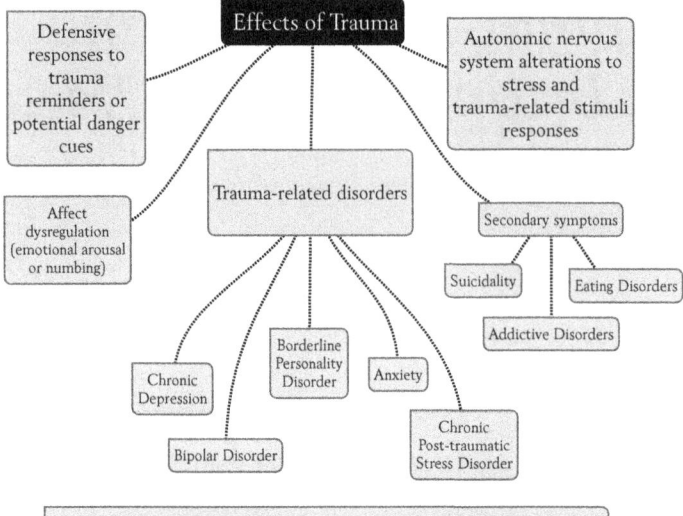

Effects of Trauma

- Defensive responses to trauma reminders or potential danger cues
- Autonomic nervous system alterations to stress and trauma-related stimuli responses
- Affect dysregulation (emotional arousal or numbing)
- Trauma-related disorders
  - Chronic Depression
  - Bipolar Disorder
  - Borderline Personality Disorder
  - Anxiety
  - Chronic Post-traumatic Stress Disorder
- Secondary symptoms
  - Suicidality
  - Eating Disorders
  - Addictive Disorders

Fisher, J. (2011). Sensorimotor approaches to trauma treatment. Advances in Psychiatric Treatment, 17(3), 171-177. doi:10.1192/apt.bp.109.007054

Before we go too deep, consider a wide-angle view as context for the work ahead. While it's not my intention to overwhelm you on the first page of this section, this Effects of Trauma mind map is a mind-blower. This overview shows us how the pieces of trauma research connect. The body of work on this topic is a critical piece of the story.

> *"Trauma is not just an event that took place sometime in the past; it is also the imprint left by that experience on mind, brain, and body. This imprint has ongoing consequences for how the human organism manages to survive in the present."*
> -Bessel van der Kolk MD[39]

The story of Compassionate Recovery began by order of importance with the story of ACEs. The story of ACEs is the story of toxic stress. What happens on a physical, brain level in toxic stress is the next step in this story of healing? Let me tell you why this is important.

Healing is only enhanced through the understanding of what goes on with us. Imagine if you were a princess, unable to sleep night after night until diagnosed with a Sleep Deprivation Disorder! Thinking that a new purple mattress would probably help, you discovered that there was a pea under your old mattress! That would be an example of an underlying impediment to your beauty sleep—not that you need it; you look fantastic—that you'd probably want to be aware of.

We can go to the doctor and demand a pill for our headache, or we can listen, and maybe she'll inform us that we have a tension headache that can be

---

[39] The Body Keeps the Score: Brain, Mind, and Body in the Healing of Trauma

relieved at home. In most people, it's caused by stress[40]. If we reduce the stress, we reduce some effects of stress, not just the headache. Other considerations could include behavioral changes such as improved ergonomics, reduced caffeine, and more reasonable work deadlines. All of these can be managed. We can do some foam rolling, take more walks, and get a massage to find relief—instead of a pill. If we learn about the cause, it makes applying a solution easier.

The first medicine we apply is that of awareness on the deepest core wounds affected by our ACEs and addictions. So far, you've explored whether or not you're on the ACEs spectrum and, if so, where. Hopefully, that knowledge means something to you personally. You're conversant—maybe more than some clinicians—on the long-term impacts of ACEs on the attachment-addiction spectrum. You've had a heads up on signposts to be aware of if you have ACEs and are in recovery as you draw your roadmap of recovery. There will be more of these up ahead.

The mission of this section is to cover just enough brain information about what happens in trauma and addiction to get a feeling for it in ourselves. You'll know how to check in with yourself and your support system with an overview and an action plan for when triggers or backdraft happen. You'll learn about what is happening and have some training in

---

[40] https://www.mayoclinic.org

circumventing stress responses that could otherwise send you down a nasty spiral on any or all the four dimensions; physical, mental, emotional, and spiritual.

You won't have to memorize brain anatomy. But you will get a sense of the mechanisms and circuitries affected by toxic stress and addiction. It's a must to understand how the pieces fit, but not necessarily the terms and jargon. What follows may be an oversimplification. The field is vast, complex, and filled with specialists with particular areas of focus. I'm not one of them. But with the help of some generous researchers who spent time with me, I think the essential points can be made clear for our needs. What are our purposes in studying the brain?

We need to understand what happens in our bodies regarding addiction and recovery. We are adding ACEs as a necessary part of the story. They offer a framework for understanding our common humanity on the attachment-addiction spectrum. What does that mean?

No matter where we are on any spectrum or our object of attachment, we can see that we have more in common with others than we thought. As this awareness deepens, it will help reduce the pervasive stress in our system that comes from feeling different.

The subsequent issues make recovery a challenge for even the sincerest among us. This kind of layout of recovery isn't what was available to me when I returned from relapse. This is what I wish was available back then. We can see the overview and choose where we need to focus on the close-in work that's part of our plan regardless of our background, position on the attachment-addiction spectrum, or anything else. You don't have to work on your trauma in your first months or even years of recovery. It's great if you can, but the idea here is to give you some ideas to support you wherever you are, rather than telling you that you must follow Step One, Step Two, Step Three in order in a precise way. This is much more on you to customize and take responsibility for your experiences and impact on others.

The idea isn't to become some sort of Brain Brainiac unless that's your thing, but to give you enough working brain knowledge to understand and explain the key points of trauma and addiction's impact. Then you'll understand what it takes to create a healing effect in the same areas of the brain in the same stress system. This will be necessary to benefit from the things you're invited to do in Compassionate Recovery. Our brains have different parts for different things. Some of it gets impaired in ACE survivors. The parts that get impaired and the chemicals involved affect many important aspects of our health and ability to function, let alone thrive.

The critical piece that we need to grasp is the common denominator between the effects on the brain from trauma and those from addiction. Other factors are more affected by trauma, and some are more affected by addiction. To understand the relationship between the systems affected by trauma and those affected by addiction, we need to find the common denominators.

Chapter 5
The Spectrum of Stress

"No matter how happy you are, you can wake up one day without any specific thing occurring to bring you into a darker place, and you'll just be in a darker place anyway."
— Chris Cornell

Everybody knows what stress is, but fewer understand the degrees of stress and the impact as we ratchet up the stress levels. According to Dr. George F. Koob, a significant figure in addiction brain research,

"Stress can be classically defined as the nonspecific (common) result of any demand upon the body or, from a more psychological perspective, anything which causes an alteration of psychological homeostatic processes.[41]"

Simply put, stress can be any change that requires a response in the body. The ability of our system to maintain stability during stress is called allostasis.

---

[41] Koob G. F. (2015). The darkness within: individual differences in stress. Cerebrum : the Dana forum on brain science, 2015, 4.

Most addicts would admit that any change is almost always stressful! But we do have everyday stresses that don't typically have negative long-term health consequences.

Normal Stress

At the beginning of the Spectrum of Stress is Eustress, the term for normal, positive stress. It is necessary for healthy development because the brain needs to learn appropriate responses to everyday stressors as it builds. Normal stress occurs when you go for a run, apply for a job, or meet your new flame. Some people seek even more of it with more thrill-seeking such as roller coasters and sky diving. This kind of stress is fun. It takes us past our limits, and out of it, we get refreshed.

Do not compare yourself with others on what it means to be normal! Your normal stress baseline may differ from others due to many factors. It's important to note that the term normal means any stress that is normal for you and doesn't throw you outside of your window of tolerance for stress.

For example, I went to a meditation retreat. Everyone else was what I call a regulated person. Someone stepped in my path and told me what I was doing wrong. Since my heart was open for the meditation practice, their aggression pierced to the core of my limbic system and sent me into an allostatic overload. I was way outside my window of tolerance while everyone else was fine. It took a couple of days to get regulated after that experience because I went into overdrive and couldn't come down. My heart was racing, and my thoughts were on fire. Because of the practices of compassion, I knew what was happening and what to do. I left the retreat and participated at home by Zoom. It was safer for me, and I was able to regulate. But if I didn't understand what was happening, that could've set me up for a spiral into the funnel or worse.

Integration Practice: Fun Stress

Make a list of some examples of positive stress you have in your life. Attachments and addictions aren't examples of positive stress because, by definition, they're problematic. Any events, past, present, or things you'd like to try can go on the list. That's the integration part of the exercise. Add one new positive stress activity, such as cardio exercises from fast walking to jumping jacks. You decide. Start anywhere. Commit to something achievable, such as one hour per week of basketball. Increase any amount. It'll be fantastic. For a Field Practice, try Fun Stress with Friends!

Tolerable Stress

The next level on the spectrum is Episodic or Acute Stress. This enters the space of Distress on our spectrum. It's temporary, event-related stress from ordinary losses, such as an unexpected job change or an illness. It's the stress level that you can move on from even if it rocks you for a bit. There are no serious long-term effects to be expected unless the stress continues.

Toxic Stress

If there is little or no relief from the stressful situation and no support, it becomes Chronic or Enduring stress. We can apply this knowledge right now. Here's how. If you're stressing out, get some help and try to give yourself a break.

Integration Practice: Calm in Your Palm

Before you begin, find stillness with a straight back and feet on the floor for grounding. Note to yourself that this can be a trigger area. Where in your body is the calm state of mind?[42] Put your palm or awareness there to enhance it. Feel the warmth exchange and the ocean of stillness growing. You are inside it. Find the ground beneath your feet. Notice the subtle movement of breath. If you find your heart racing, notice the pulsing of your heart. Relax and observe the experience, nice and easy.

Whenever you feel stress, remember the calm in your palm. Now that you're chill af, list some of the most salient episodes of acute yet tolerable stress in your life. As you write the details at whatever level

---

[42] If the answer isn't obvious, it's OK. Imagine your body as a vast ocean, with a perfectly still floor.

you wish, notice the sensations in the body. Keep the calm palm handy.

When the Episodic becomes the Chronic, it is the beginning of what is referred to in addiction and psychological trauma literature as Toxic Stress. When we can't get a break from the stress overload, and there's no one to help us—as helpless children—our brain's ability to regulate stress becomes partly disabled. The circuits responsible for emotional regulation and the neurotransmitters that connect those circuits can be inhibited. Those inhibitions create wiring changes to the brain circuits due in part to Allostatic Overload. If we get to this point, we don't regulate the stress. Stress regulates us.

Allostatic Load

In Fall 2020, Jenny Guidi and her team at the Department of Psychology, University of Bologna, were stuck in the lockdown in Italy. They decided to use the downtime to review over 500 scientific journal articles on Allostatic Load and Overload before they refined the focus to the 267 most significant. They wanted to summarize the complete knowledge on this topic to make informed recommendations to clinicians who treat people like us. From their metanalysis,

"Allostatic load refers to **the cumulative burden of chronic stress and life events**. ... When environmental challenges exceed the individual ability to cope, then allostatic overload ensues.[43]"

They found that early life traumas predicted allostatic overload outcomes such as Post Traumatic Stress Syndrome or PTSD, discussed in Chapter 11. These findings give you what you need to know from the current literature on Allostatic Load (AL). The following are considered predictors of high AL. It means that there's a strong chance if you have something on this list, that you'll experience overload.

- Low socioeconomic status.
- Ethnicity is a factor, with blacks more likely than whites to have high levels of AL.
- New immigrants
- Perceived racial discrimination
- Social inequality
- Race discrimination
- Weight discrimination
- Gender-related characteristics such as being androgynous, undifferentiated, or non-masculine
- Sexual orientation; lesbian, gay, bisexual
- Feeling we have less physical or mental skills

---

[43] Guidi J, Lucente M, Sonino N, Fava G, A: Allostatic Load and Its Impact on Health: A Systematic Review. Psychother Psychosom 2021;90:11-27. doi: 10.1159/000510696

As we can expect, ACEs also made the list because they lead to high AL. Those with high overload have sleep problems, bad diets, are overweight, and consume too much alcohol and cigarettes. We have a higher chance for heart disease, poor psychosocial functioning, high rates of psychopathology, psychological distress such as anxiety and depressive disorders, lower well-being, and impaired quality of life. For alcoholics, relapse severity and post-treatment drinking were related to high AL going into treatment and increased AL due to life stressors and the inability to manage in recovery after treatment. When we're on the wrong end of the spiral, the worse it gets, the worse it gets.

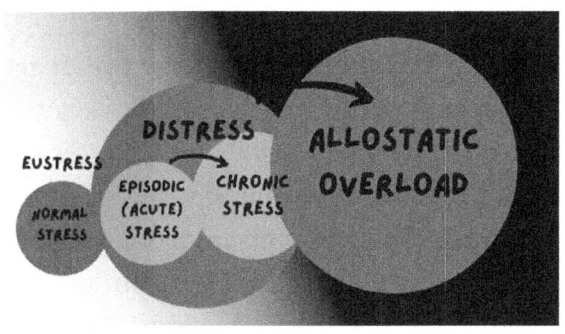

[Diagram: Nested circles labeled NORMAL STRESS (inside EUSTRESS), EPISODIC (ACUTE) STRESS and CHRONIC STRESS (inside DISTRESS), with an arrow pointing to ALLOSTATIC OVERLOAD]

But what are the factors that predict lower Allostatic Load? AL can get higher as we get older, particularly if we lose cognitive and physical function. But the good news is that people with dogs have lower AL than people without dogs.[44]

Here's a big one: perceived social support. People need people. Things like warmth in the home and parental involvement in school are *reverse* indicators of AL. The more support we feel we have, the more we can chill on the lower end of our stress spectrum. It's easy to see why a caring significant other makes such a substantial impact on kids experiencing ACEs and why community-based support groups are so beneficial. We will also have a plan to get out of a triggering situation that includes a support system. We'll talk about building a Circle of Safety coming up.

Other things that decrease AL are when we have meaning and purpose in our lives. Meaning-making is a big deal for our recovery. Physical activity

---

[44] You hear that David Sedaris?

lightens our load. Remember, getting the heart rate up for 20 minutes a day, for example, is beneficial for stress.

Dr. Guidi's review recommendations indicate that a multi-disciplinary approach is needed to address these toxic stress issues. Additionally, they recommend healthy lifestyle changes. The practices in this book are designed to create changes that reduce the load on our systems. It only works if you do the work. So, we do the work. Say it right now, "I'm doing the work!"

With all of this in mind, it makes sense that as we learn to relax and be at ease with ourselves on all our physical, mental, emotional, and spiritual levels, it will lower our Allostatic Load. Something essential for our recovery toolbox is knowing how to keep the load low by staying within our functional comfort zone, called the Window of Tolerance.

Notes

Chapter 6
The Window of Tolerance

"Everyone you meet is fighting a battle you know nothing about. Be kind. Always."
– Robin Williams

Our nervous system needs to be calm in order to reboot our brain circuits after living with the effects of toxic stress. But our brains and bodies are designed to seek, not to be still. We must move forward to get our basic needs met. Food doesn't drop out of the sky. When they're not, our nervous systems don't relax. If we can't relax when we're distressed and don't have a way to regulate, we're at the mercy of the triggering situation. We must survive it until the stimulation dies down and we eventually return to baseline. But if there's no way to be at baseline before an allostatic meltdown, we can expect instability and dysregulation.

If you have an ACE score, think about yourself trying to do well in school after extreme abuse or neglect at home. Did you learn to be calm when distressed? Did you react to the overload by getting addicted to drugs or cutting school in an unwitting effort to manage a system impaired by toxic stress? Kids like us grow up to have a very narrow window of tolerance. The norm was to get triggered and spiral into highs and lows that made everything worse. And all of it would have a long-term impact on our quality of life.

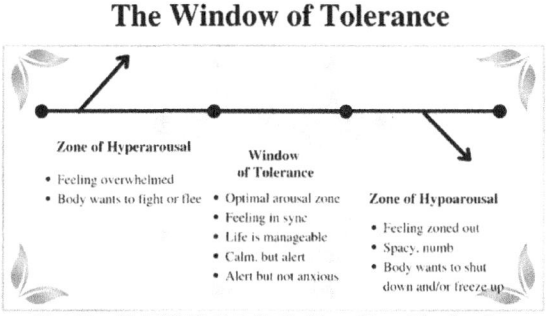

The Window of Tolerance

Zone of Hyperarousal
- Feeling overwhelmed
- Body wants to fight or flee

Window of Tolerance
- Optimal arousal zone
- Feeling in sync
- Life is manageable
- Calm, but alert
- Alert but not anxious

Zone of Hypoarousal
- Feeling zoned out
- Spacy, numb
- Body wants to shut down and/or freeze up

Adapted from Seigel (2009) Mindsight - The New Science of Personal Transformation

We can expand our window of tolerance and learn to regulate, no matter what our ACE score is or how far we traveled into the attachment-addiction spectrum. We can and must rewrite our mental scripts into new narratives based on principles and practices of compassion.

If you're early in recovery, knowing about your Window of Toleranceis especially to your benefit. You'll have a baseline to refer to throughout your recovery. Wherever we are on the recovery-mastery spectrum, we can benefit from knowing how to read the signals on all our dimensions that would possibly trigger us into The Funnel.

Dr. Dan Siegel, Clinical Professor of Psychiatry at the School of Medicine of the University of

California, Los Angeles, described the Window of Tolerance to understand and describe normal brain and body reactions, particularly in the wake of ACEs. We can have any of these states in general or more specific ways. The various windows we have each live in their spectrum, but our whole system is affected at any given moment.

Where is your window of tolerance right now on the following? Add other dimensions that come up for you.

Anger
I feel nothing.
I'm angry, but it's not getting in the way.
I'm getting pretty riled up right about now!

Sadness
I feel buried in sorrow or grief.
I'm sad, but I can function alright.
I'm sobbing and hyperventilating.

Peace
I feel like I don't even know what the word means.
I'm alright, chill af. No problems. All good atm.
I'm so peaced-out got zero fux to give. Beach day!

The first emotional state in each of the above examples indicates hypoarousal. Hypoarousal, according to complextrauma.org, is the state beneath our Window of Tolerance where we feel low, emotionally dead, and can barely function. We don't want to connect with others or even care for our bodies. Hypoarousal can be triggered by painful memories or feelings, lack of stimulation, and real or imagined threats.

Think about some times when you've been emotionally in a state of hypoarousal. If the words don't come, pull out the breakup playlist. If you don't have a sad and rainy-day list of songs, make one. Where in the body do you feel the least sensation when you're hypoaroused? How do you sleep? What are your eating habits at those times? What attachments or addictions do you turn to?

These are some of the ways we adapt to our states. Sometimes these behavioral adaptations are alright, but as many of us familiar with the dark underbelly of tolerance know, it's easy to understand why we'd choose to fight the downside with stimulants like sugar, caffeine, or methamphetamine. Don't worry. These adaptations can be replaced with new, intentional ones. That's what this work is about.

The second statement of the examples is a window where we feel functional. As we alluded to earlier, this can be an elusive experience. But we can train ourselves over time to identify our dysregulation and take actions to regulate ourselves. There would be no reason for this book if that weren't possible.

We can learn to Drop into a window of tolerance. Imagine a pond, in the middle of a forest, with no ripples. Sit like this for some time, without moving but relaxed and supple. Be the pond. You are the pond, and some fish swim by. The movement in stillness caused by the energy of the fishes doesn't disturb you. You're settled and calm. You are the fishes, swimming gracefully through the still waters.

Where were you when you last felt like you were within your window on some emotion or overall? What times of the day do you get the most done? When are you the least functional? How are you with your window of sleep? These things give you a baseline for your current windows on different dimensions.

When you identify with the third question, you're looking at a state of hyperarousal. From our excellent resource earlier, [45] hyperarousal is where our physiology is overloaded; our emotions are peaking and frying our circuits. We're hypersensitive and overreactive and have a high chance of becoming aggressive or violent. Some of us learn to adapt by keeping ourselves jacked up in a hyper-aroused state. We can be stress junkies, crisis addicts, and toxic relationship-aholics—whatever keeps us trippin' and feeling at home in a state of dysregulation.

When was the last time you made a social media post in a state of hyperarousal? What holiday is the most shame-inducing for you to remember? Did you look back months or years later and have no idea who would say or do something like that? We all have. You're not alone. This is part of life's suffering.

---

45 www.complextrauma.org/glossary/

Learning about it will help develop deep compassion for self and others.

Write down three examples of being agitated, overexcited, and charged up to the point of losing your ability to think clearly and make rational decisions based on self-compassion. What windows were you out of when you were in those states? Take these questions seriously, regardless of how long it takes to get clarity. It will come, I promise. Have conversations with other people in recovery about this topic. Over time we learn together.

Learning to check in with ourselves and each other when we experience dysregulation is key to understanding how to be OK without our attachments and addictions.

Understanding your window of tolerance will help you have more tolerance of other people's window of tolerance. Tolerance means we handle the intensity. If we lose functionality somehow, we're falling outside of our window of tolerance. Stress can put us into a depressive spiral or a manic episode. We all know of people who do better in stressful times and even seek thrills, while others are overwhelmed by excitement. Intensity from outside ourselves or our internal self-defeating narratives affects how we think, feel and act. It can be tricky because sometimes we don't know we're outside our tolerance until we've gone too far, such as an angry outburst. If we're not used to being still enough in our bodies to notice our emotional energy, we may not know that we are getting angry until somebody's flat on their ass and we're in handcuffs.

It's common that addicts and the otherwise traumatized struggle with identifying and experiencing feelings. For example, I phone-dated a girl during the pandemic who had no answer whenever I asked her how she felt. Silence. Why don't you answer? I'm not used to being asked this question. I don't know how I feel, but I'm trying to learn. My friend didn't know how to identify her feelings, so she didn't know how to answer. The part that hit me was when she said, "I'm not used to people asking me that." I had no answer for that. All I feel is feelings, all the time. It's the real reason I drank and drugged myself, nearly to death at times in my life.

What happens when we fall out of tolerance? A surge of emotions can flood us mentally and disrupt our ability to reason and act normally. It means a breakdown, a relapse, or a scene at home or work for some of us. It's not hard to make the connection here that addicts, the traumatized, those with PTSD and related disorders can be triggered by intense experiences, internally or externally, that throw them out of tolerance.

When we suffer from trauma, we can lose the ability to self-regulate, making our Window of Tolerance smaller. By definition, it is difficult to get into the comfort zone if we are over or under-stimulated. We're easily triggered and usually have no idea what's happening with us. As our episodes of out-of-control behavior stack up, the layers of shame get deeper. Our alienation grows, and our sense of personal agency shrinks. It's effortless to get addicted while seeking relief from these unbearable states. However, it seems like we're controlling something in addiction, but ultimately it controls us. We, therefore, must find a way to be in recovery and do the deep healing to keep us in recovery. We want to be growing and fresh, not stale and jaded. If we don't do the work, we might turn into one of those bitter old farts in recovery, pointing a crooked finger and hissing at newcomers.

The practices here can widen our Window of Tolerance, but we may also need to manage our triggers with professional help. Remember, backdraft happens. There are many clinicians skilled in this concept. You might be wise to seek a clinician to help with this process. To function better, we need to widen the window in ways that we can tolerate.

A wider window means we can handle the intensity. That gives us a better chance to stay on the recovery-mastery spectrum and develop ourselves into the person we've always wanted to be. If we understand and monitor our Window of Tolerance, we'll become more tolerant.

Integration Practice: Be a Big Window

Sit in a room with three different aspects of yourself. You're all on comfortable chairs facing a small window. What do each of you see? Describe what is seen through the tiny window one by one, from the perspective of each of these aspects. Be like an actor and change character for each description. Below are some examples. Try to come up with your own versions of these questions as a general life awareness practice that allows the light of compassion to shine throughout the day's activities. Fill in the blanks with what comes up for you. Return to this exercise at different points in your recovery. Note dates in your journal.

Who am I right now?

I am the aspect of self that is on the conservative side. I see the need for things to be…
My view is limited to my belief structure. Things are the way they are, and that is that.

I'm the aspect of self that's more liberal. I see everything as an opportunity for…
My view is limited to my belief structure. Things are the way they are, and that is that.
I'm the aspect of self that lives in the flow state. I resist nothing, and everything falls into place. It's

like magic. Intuition works, ideas flow, and problems get solved.

All three of these aspects sit as one, looking out the same window. Imagine that it's much bigger. You can see the broader view with these integrated aspects. It requires discernment but gives your focus a finely sharpened edge. Finish the rest of the exercise in your own words. How do things look now, through this expanded window of inner perceptions? Use a lot of paint or colored crayons to answer. Yes, you can do the melty kind; just be safe!

The Big Window practice lets you open your windows of tolerance considerably more, especially when you learn to reflect this tolerance to others in the community. Learn to have deep compassion for all your Windows of Tolerance. They are the way they are for a good reason. You are currently healing. This is a good thing. As soon as you see the opportunity, bring Wisdom from this work into the world. Talk to friends about it. That kind of mission will keep you sober if you know your Window of Tolerance limitations and how to realistically work on opening them wider.

Now that we know what the Window of Tolerance is and how it works in our own lives let's look more deeply into how the Window of Tolerance functions in the body. It's all based on our nervous system. It's helpful to be aware of how we're built and function. But don't let the content make you nervous!

Notes

Chapter 7
The Nervous System

"Dearly beloved, we are gathered here today to get through this thing called life."
— Prince

Ancient teachings, as well as cognitive psychology, tell us that we are the architects of our experience. Yet when we're out of tolerance, we don't feel like we have direct control over our emotional experiences. That is because the nervous system gets dysregulated, and we fall out our window of tolerance on one dimension or another. Here's some amazing news. Once we know about it and apply contextualized practices that help us regulate, many significant changes in our perceptions and experiences occur. An integrated recovery roadmap that includes methods like yoga, martial arts, cardio bursts, and other movements, combined with seated meditation, can teach us to regulate. Our physical, emotional, mental, and spiritual energy states can be regulated by doing things that affect our main regulatory system, the ANS or Autonomic Nervous System. The ANS is made up of two branches that regulate internal physical processes like heart rate, breathing, blood pressure, body temperature, digestion, sexual response, pupil dilation, the pitch of your voice, and the rate at which you speak salivation, and swallowing. They work together and separately, such as during sex, where excitement and a chill vibe happen simultaneously. After all, nobody wants a parasympathetic partner.

Although the ANS operates without us having to tell it to, the fact that it's automatic doesn't stop us from changing our nervous system with our practice and our intention to heal.

There are volumes on the relationship between our emotional regulation and our ability to do something about it when we need to. What you need to know is that the activities such as those mentioned above are a vital part of your recovery toolbox. Get into mind-body movement ASAP. Go into a quiet space. Put on old songs, soft and emotive. Close your eyes and move effortlessly until you simply complete the movement. Then be very still for some time.

Sympathetic Nervous System

The SNS branch is named so because it is sympathetic and responsive to your feelings.[46] In Greek, "syn" means co, or synthesis and working

---

[46] Please don't suggest to your partner that they need to be more like your SNS.

together with our emotions. The SNS uses norepinephrine to create a stimulating response. Now I don't want anybody gettin' trigger happy. Still, the sympathetic system is responsible for all that fight or flight stress hormone jacking up that can happen when real or imagined terrible and fantastic things occur or do not occur. To some of our brains, the thing being right there in front of us or not is irrelevant. When triggered by internal, external, real, or conditioned memories or sensations, the internal stress response will be the same as if the Wholly Mammoth were right there, fangs dripping with whatever foamy stuff they spewed back in the Pleistocene landscape.

We get the heart contractions; eyeballs dilate like we're rolling on Molly at an ODESZA concert, our sweaty leg muscles ready to respond. Suppose we don't wet ourselves when whatever our six ton eleven-foot-high thing triggers us. In that case, we'll forget about peeing, and our digestion will stop because those processes are superseded by the body's perceived need to GTFO[47].

The ACE'd out among us usually have no idea why we're dropping out of windows left and right. Even though we're trying to spiral upward instead of downward into the funnel of attachment and addiction, panic attacks, anxiety, and depression feel like they're forever holding us back. That's

---

47 Get The Fuck Out!

because we didn't understand the simplicity of regulating our systems. The automatic part of the autonomic nervous system kicks stress hormones into high gear. How can we possibly have known this? Doctors toss pills at us, and everyone else throws their hands in the air.

These processes are not going to hold you back anymore. Because the work is right here, and the work will set you free. Do the work.

Insight Practice: What's Your Woolly Mammoth?

Real people, places, and things trigger our nervous systems to go into Allostatic Overload, causing Toxic Stress that drives our addictions. Make a table of these by categories, such as type of person, common situation, or a place that has sent your ANS into Hyperarousal. Next, rewrite the narrative into a fantastic story. Write out the kind of qualities and skills that you might need if you were to overcome these triggers. Use your imagination.

Begin writing a story about an aspect of yourself that learns to ride the "Woolly Mammoth." Yours can be any creature or image representing one of those people, places, or crazy things that make you crazy. But in this story, you create a scenario where the hero walks away with the prize. Remember, stories have a beginning, a middle, and an end.

There's conflict, struggle, and near-death, and eventually, the hero gets on the horse because he couldn't find a Mammoth.

For extra credit, redeemable by peace and wisdom points, read your story aloud to a person or a dog. If you don't feel comfortable writing a story, you may substitute by creating a rap jam by rewriting the lyrics to the same beat as your favorite Golden Era joint. But you will have to rap it down at the next Bar Mitzvah you're invited to.

Parasympathetic Nervous System

Our Parasympathetic (PNS) branch of the ANS uses the neurotransmitter acetylcholine to stimulate resting and digesting. A full belly and a good couch where we'd like to be! But if we're in a hypomanic swing out of our Window of Tolerance, we may need to exercise to give ourselves energy when in a low parasympathetic state.

The parasympathetic [48] controls body process during our ordinary activities. Its function is to conserve and restore energy by slowing the heart rate and decreasing blood pressure. It also regulates digestive energy so we can process food and have those good, S-shaped poops that were all the rave on Oprah.

---

48 https://www.merckmanuals.com/

It's easy for anyone [49] to feel the difference between the sympathetic and parasympathetic systems. Want to try it? Great!

Breath in. You just activated the sympathetic system, which then switches on the neurotransmitter adrenaline, that in turn causes an increase in your heart rate.

Ok, you can breathe out now. Boom, parasympathetic slowdown of heart rate brings us back to resting. In Hot Yoga class, we lie down motionless on our backs for one minute. Then we resume the intensely brutal practice. Given what you've learned, why do you think that happens?

Since we spend so much time stuck in fight or flight, it makes sense to learn how to get out of that adrenaline response when we need to get into some acetylcholine chill-out time.

Integration Practice: What Goes Up Must Come Down

The trick is to increase your heart rate for a short period, followed by a very short rest. Then two more rounds. You can do Football Runners, Jumping Jacks, High Knee Raises, Running in Place, or even mindful walking if it gets your heart rate up. If those are unfamiliar terms, get on yer Google and watch

---

49 Caveat, you must be alive.

the Youtubes. Subscribe and like your favorites. Do their classes with friends and family, lovers[50] and other strangers? But the key is to bring it up, rest a little, repeat. Do that routine three times per set. Work up to more sets and more exercises. Make it super fun. Engage a friend in this activity. Call it "working out to regulate your mood, so you don't reach for your attachments." Who's going to say no to an offer like that?

Here's an example.

Jump up and down with moderate effort for one minute.

Set your timer for 20 seconds.

Jump up and down as fast as you safely can for 20 seconds. Remember, that's 20 whole seconds, not 19 seconds.

Rest for 10 seconds. Not 11 seconds.

Do two more rounds.

Each round of 20 seconds is maximum effort. This will vary for all kinds of different bodies and experiences. For some, what looks light may get the heart rate up quickly. For others, it takes a mountain. Learn what you need in your physical dimension because tending and training your heart and lungs is part of the path of recovery. The good news is that you can start where you are. Consistency is key. Practice is dose-related. Will you become a workout junkie and run 100-milers? Some

---

[50] and other strangers

do. I began with ten-minute walks around the block and eventually became a yoga and fitness instructor. So just start. Now. Let it take you where it takes you.

If you have doubts or medical concerns, please consult a personal trainer. However, I have confidence that you won't harm yourself if you learn how to do this kind of interval training. It's good. Real good. It's the best thing ever. I taught it for a decade to thousands of students. Once you learn the benefits of interval training as a tool for recovery, you'll never want to let a day pass without it. It's the best way to regulate your nervous system if you combine it with meditation and other good things like that. Here's how.

You bring up the intensity with exercise, then bring it back down with self-soothing practices, contemplative activities, meditations, yoga, mindful music, or anything that chills you out. I've had friends who could only chill out to Death Metal. Learn your system. Give yourself what you need like one of my yoga students did.

Jan was 27, a graduate student in chemistry at the University of Arizona. They had a hard time in class, so they utilized the university's counseling center for support. This got them through college, but even years after graduation, they felt the same underlying anxiety they had under the pressure of being in graduate school. Back then, they struggled with Adderall abuse, at first during finals but developing into a severe problem. Jan was rockin' it on all levels in their work and career, yet unable to manage any serious relationship and had severe bouts of depression and loneliness.

They were discouraged that after doing personal work for so long, there were still so many challenges. After years of attacking life's problems with hard work, Jan took up Power Yoga [51], emphasizing core strength and cardio activity. Through the practice, they realized that pushing hard wasn't always the solution. Jan started coming to class early to meditate and learned to relax more than they'd ever been able to before. Yet they also found that the experience of working with their body opened emotions that were confusing and difficult. After several months of combining somatic trauma work with a trained therapist and yoga, Jan understood that they had a viewpoint that everything could be solved by banging away at it with a work ethic. This subconscious perspective had been a positive motivation toward success, but it was also an inhibiting factor to health and wellbeing. It took a lot of hard work, but Jan eventually grew from getting at that stuck point and was able to go in some new directions as a result.

The cycle of addiction deepens the grooves of trauma, and as we'll see, that works in reverse. Trauma makes addiction worse. Addiction makes itself worse, which is trauma. The cycle is toxic and

---

[51] http://poweryoga.com

deadly. This is a vital point to understand. If you have this understanding, it will strengthen your recovery. The self-compassion that we learn and practice in this book gives us the power to choose the path for ourselves when it matters most. There comes a crucial moment in our addiction when we can turn left and die or turn right and GTFO. What's it going to be?

It comes down to picking up our addictions or choosing to do hard things that nurture us on the deepest levels. The work is like the six root canals I had in Mexico this winter. To heal the sickness, we get down to the core where the sickness of past trauma lives. A teacher once said that the issues live in our tissues.

When this kind of information sinks in, actions that cause self-harm start to feel foreign and toxic, like big ugly turds floating in a newly built crystal blue swimming pool of compassion and wisdom.

Wouldn't it be nicer to swim in fresh, clean water? Let's learn about what flips our switches next so we can put the next part of the story together.

Notes

Chapter 8
Neurotransmitters

*"All the other kids with the pumped-up kicks
You better run, better run,
outrun my gun
All the other kids with the pumped-up kicks
You better run, better run
faster than my bullet"*
-Mark Foster[52]

Now that we have what we need to know about the mechanisms of toxic stress and how it affects our nervous system's window of tolerance, let's narrow the focus down to the level of neurotransmitters (NTs). We briefly mentioned two, norepinephrine and acetylcholine, in the last chapter. We need to understand a few more building blocks to tell the rest of the story. The good news is that this brief discussion is as granular as we'll get, and it will be enough.

This kind of detail doesn't need to be memorized. It's sufficient to get a sense of how it works. That's all

---

[52] Songwriters: Mark Foster, Foster the People, Pumped Up Kicks lyrics © Notting Hill Music UK Limited

you need to know to *make meaning* of the solutions we apply here. Doing empty practices like some kind of Zen Zombie probably doesn't do much healing for us. The more we study, the deeper we learn and the more we know. With deep knowledge, we can access and apply healing methods to the subterranean places where it hurts. Knowledge of this sort doesn't need to be an intellectual process. In fact, it's more effective in a felt sense rather than a thinking sense.

When we Drop into our meditations, we have a headlamp to guide us. Think of this brain stuff as your headlamp to self-compassion. When we understand what's happening with us, we can feel compassion. After deepening this knowledge into our guts and bones, we will have a much more healing effect on others than before. It's amazing. I hope you'll do the work to get the benefits.

You'll recall our discussion on the fight, flight, or freeze responses. Neurotransmitters are the chemical messengers that turn on these responses in the complex brain network of circuitries.[53] For simplicity, let's think of NTs as on/off switches in these circuitries. Adrenaline, for example, is a switch that turns on and off hundreds of billions of times per second, depending on what's happening—or what we perceive is happening. When switched

---

[53] A circuit is a closed energy system. Circuitries are systems made up of circuits that perform particular functions, such as the drive to seek a tasty cheeseburger.

on, NTs connect to a circuit telling the body what to do, like jump out of the path of a charging Woolly Mammoth. That's all well and good, as long as there's a Wholly Mammoth. If there's no threat, and our adrenaline switch is stuck in the always-on position, we're on track for toxic stress and all of the implications we've discussed.

In summary, stress is the response to changes in the environment. NTs are what make that response happen in our ANS and other systems. Toxic stress from ongoing trauma causes what some researchers call a "distorted cascade" of neurotransmitters. This jacks our Allostatic Load and puts us at risk on all four dimensions in the short and the long term. For this reason, it's necessary to know a few terms so we can have an informed discussion of what this means to us on the path of recovery, particularly for those of us with ACEs.

Catecholamines

The catecholamines are the group of NTs that support how our bodies respond to stress. When you cross the street and realize there's a bus coming straight at you, this group of NTs switches on, giving you what you need to GTFO of the way and save your skin.

The adrenal glands produce the catecholamines that you need to know. Epinephrine (adrenaline), norepinephrine (noradrenaline), and dopamine. What do they do?

- increase heart rate
- raise blood pressure
- ramp up breathing rate
- blast muscle strength
- sharpen mental alertness
- lower blood flow to the skin and guts, which are not necessary for immediate survival
- increase bow flow to the more organs essential to sustain life: the brain, heart, and kidneys[54]

Catecholamines function correctly when all our dimensions of being human are doing what they are supposed to do. As we'll see, toxic stress changes the balance significantly. When we're out of our window of tolerance on something like emotional anger, we might have a hard time slowing down the stress before it jacks us up to a place where we don't want to be. We're talking about this because we can understand the problems and apply fantastic solutions that will do good things for our humanness.

---

[54] https://www.uofmhealth.org/health-library/tw12861

Let's go through these so that later when we talk about the bigger systems, it will be very clear. This list is not exhaustive. Like everything else in this section, it's a reduction of a vast amount of complex material to what is directly relevant to our compassionate healing.

Epinephrin\Adrenaline

Epinephrin alerts your system to go into overdrive immediately upon sensing a threat. For addicts, it's easy to over-identify with this temporary surge of power. If we're out of balance, a surge of it can put us in a precarious place where we can't make good decisions.

Norepinephrine\Noradrenaline

Levels of norepinephrine increase during a stress response. Consistent with the other catecholamines, this NT shifts the blood flow to the right places to get us where we need to be gettn' to real quick-like.

Dopamine

A neurotransmitter that has to do with reward and punishment, pleasure and pain, dopamine, or DA, is probably the most famous one next to adrenaline. I can't remember a yoga class where the instructor didn't remind us that we were "making dopamine" and were going to feel great! It was no lie. I spent over a decade taking and teaching yoga. We deliberately manufactured adrenaline with high-intensity interval training in my classes, then brought it down with a slower, more dopamine-inducing practice. There are ways to control these neurotransmitters that affect us so profoundly.

Did I mention that fitness is key to recovery because it's key to physical, mental, and emotional health? Start today. You won't regret it.

Most people have heard that dopamine makes us feel better. It does, and it also helps us focus. DA has different functions as it runs through eight different pathways in the brain. Dopamine's mesolimbic pathway is partly connected to the limbic or emotional system. DA will have different effects depending on which pathway and what the NT interacts with.

There are trillions of things happening at the NT level universe every instant. For this reason, we can't accurately think of dopamine as having one characteristic. What we need to know is which aspects we can use for healing.

Dopamine is also connected to physical movement, as we mentioned. But depletions of dopamine are linked to Parkinson's Disease. When DA runs through our brain's limbic system, thought to be the center of emotional processing, it affects our reward and pleasure circuitries. When we experience something that we can get attached to or addicted to, dopamine switches to the ON position and starts firing pleasurable sensations.

Dopamine motivates our brain's seeking circuitry to go-get-some! Our brains say, "Yeah, baby, I want more!" Some drugs, cocaine, nicotine, and heroin, increase the rush of dopamine, which is part of their addictive nature. The punishment-reward system in our brain is affected by addiction. Adaptations in these neural networks under the stress of continued addiction cause what researchers call behavioral abnormalities [55] and physiological changes at the substrate level. These are structural changes that can't be reversed. Don't worry; the brain can make new nerve cells. We can even create new circuits, especially if we do it with intention and a good understanding of how it works. Think about it. The power of positive thinking is energized by deliberate activities that create new dopaminergic neurons that make dopamine and are responsible for cognitive and fine motor coordination.

Deficiencies in DA are also related to sleep, dreaming, mood, attention, memory, and learning.[56] Dysregulation of dopamine pathways has been connected with several psychiatric disorders. If we have malfunctioning dopamine levels, it causes emotional disorders like depression and the

---

[55] Dianne M.A. Van den Heuvel, R. Jeroen Pasterkamp, Getting connected in the dopamine system, Progress in Neurobiology, Volume 85, Issue 1, 2008, Pages 75-93

56 Juárez Olguín, H., Calderón Guzmán, D., Hernández García, E., & Barragán Mejía, G. (2016). The Role of Dopamine and Its Dysfunction as a Consequence of Oxidative Stress. Oxidative medicine and cellular longevity, 2016, 9730467.

development of addiction. So those that are predisposed due to ACEs damage to DA systems have the compounded likelihood of developing addictive disorders.[57]

Indeed, we can intentionally change our brains. It's work, and it takes time, and we'll always have to deal with the old circuits firing up sometimes. But we can heal. That's why you're reading this, right? Because you know deep down that you can heal and want to recover. You're not alone.

Have you ever heard that recovery is an inside job? It really is.

Dynorphin

Dynorphin contributes to changes in our systems in response to stress and addiction.[58] Dynorphin is part of our opioid or internal pain management system. This stress response system controls our physical *and* emotional responses to stress and is related to addiction, schizophrenia, learning, memory, chronic pain, and depression.

It works with opioid receptors that allow the analgesic effect to take place. We've all heard that

---

[57] R. Christopher Pierce; Vidhya Kumaresan (2006). The mesolimbic dopamine system: The final common pathway for the reinforcing effect of drugs of abuse?. , 30(2), 215–238. doi:10.1016/j.neubiorev.2005.04.016

[58] Knoll, A. T., & Carlezon, W. A., Jr (2010). Dynorphin, stress, and depression. *Brain research*, *1314*, 56–73. https://doi.org/10.1016/j.brainres.2009.09.074

opiates hijack part of our natural opioid system to the point that, without the opiate, we can't tolerate even the slightest pain, emotional or physical. The opiate becomes more necessary the more necessary it becomes. Our circuitries get incredibly heightened sensitivity from this hijacking. Like other adaptations that our systems make in response to stress, trauma, and addiction, the more sensitive we get, the more sensitive we get.

MOR and DOR are two of three receptors in dynorphin. Together, they have two effects when dynorphin fires correctly under normal circumstances. First, MOR *increases* our physical ability by *decreasing* our pain sensitivity. That decreased sensitivity is due to an inhibition of pain fibers that send the message, "OW mf that hurts!" At the same time, DOR increases our motivation to escape stress by creating an unpleasant or aversive feeling that says, "Bro! Go away from this aversive and unpleasant feeling." But under long-term, acute, uncontrollable stress, adaptations occur in our neuronal functioning.

These changes in our neurological processes are called neuroadaptations, which are the result of sustained dysregulation. Neuroadaptations are the underlying condition of our addiction. They can make us more sensitive, thereby reducing our window of tolerance for alcohol and other drugs. Neuroadaptation can cause what's called counteradaptation. The systems that fire our neurotransmitters change in response to addiction. For example, we may develop a high tolerance because our system is trying to adapt to the drug by protecting itself. Withdrawal is the same process, where the body reacts to the absence of the drug and tries to adapt. Incentive salience as a response to this withdrawal stress can drop us right back down the funnel of addiction, as we know.

When the stress chemical switches are on all the time, it erodes the wiring of our circuits and can blow the network of circuitries that our brain needs to keep us whole.

The third receptor, KOR, is the primary receptor involved in that aversive state. That state, when prolonged, creates dysphoria, which is another word for depression. When the KOR system, which, if you recall, is within the neurotransmitter dynorphin, is blown out, it contributes to stress-related mood disorders.

CRF

Corticotropin-releasing factor, or CRF, is another NT with its own stress response system. The malfunctioning of CRT due to prolonged stress is like dynorphin and is related to the cause and development of mood disorders in addition to depression. Anxiety and memory issues are also on the list, along with anhedonia, the inability to feel pleasure. Anhedonia is thought to be an effect of addiction on the brain. This is why life is boring to addicts when we get sober. It's also boring to manics who are high on mania. For some of us, it's imperative to learn to get comfortable with the ordinary. The reflective, compassionate, and mindful practices in this book teach us to notice, appreciate and celebrate the ordinary.

Cortisol

Cortisol is the body's primary stress hormone. Dopamine and serotonin are also hormones in addition to being neurotransmitters. Cortisol is produced by the hypothalamus-pituitary-adrenal, or HPA axis. When too much cortisol from too much stress, dopamine and serotonin are suppressed.

Cortisol production goes up in stressful situations. The body systems that aren't necessary for immediate survival shut down, so all resources go to survival mode. If we stay at high cortisol, our brains learn to keep up that in active stress response. We adapt to high-stress situations and don't know how to feel comfortable in low-stress situations. Sound familiar?

Cortisol is part of our metabolism's ability to regulate and is important to our immune system.[59] But when the sympathetic nervous system, which you'll recall is where the fight or flight response

---

[59] Thau L, Gandhi J, Sharma S. Physiology, Cortisol. [Updated 2021 Sep 6]. In: StatPearls [Internet]. Treasure Island (FL): StatPearls Publishing; 2022 Jan-. Available from: https://www.ncbi.nlm.nih.gov/books/NBK538239/

happens, gets activated by internal or external stress, cortisol fuels it.

We haven't discussed brain parts yet, but to continue the story of cortisol, just note that it shoots down the amygdala and hits the fear trigger. If it's an acute shock of the stress transmitter, the signal travels to the hypothalamus, which kicks in the adrenal glands that blast out a cascade of catecholamines like adrenaline. That blows up the heart and breathing rate. If the situation is extreme, the hypothalamus switches on the HPA axis, and BAM! We're on high alert and ready to run like hell. Imagine being like this all the time for no apparent reason.

Serotonin

Serotonin is the neurotransmitter of happiness. It's also responsible for feelings of focus and calm. This NT is also related to bad moods. The switch gets stuck when the stress gets toxic. That's why some anti-depressants boost serotonin production. There are many complex reasons for depression. Low serotonin is part of the depression story, but it's not the whole story. Meds and exercise are among the best tools that help with serotonin-related depression problems.[60] Many drugs and addictive

---

[60] Young S. N. (2007). How to increase serotonin in the human brain without drugs. Journal of psychiatry & neuroscience : JPN, 32(6), 394–399.

behaviors cause dysregulation of serotonin and other neurotransmitters that affect every aspect of our lives.

Its helpful to know that lack of serotonin has been linked with mental health conditions, especially those relating to mood disorders and addiction. Reading about this topic may make you feel that we're chemical robots when you get down to it. To whatever extent our traumas, addictions, and other problems have been on an automatic level beyond our control, it's heavy news, but it's not the end of the story. You're only halfway through the book, after all. If there weren't something we could do about all of this, I'd have written a space novel.

Oxytocin

Though it's been popularized as the love hormone, the neurotransmitter Oxytocin can also create an experience of aggression and has been shown to enhance or supercharge anti-social behavior. It is responsible for our feelings of connection with loved ones and all phases of romantic love. We, addicts, get addicted to people. Oxytocin might as well be relationship crack for some of us. It's also part of our learning and reward systems and plays a role in pro-social behaviors and memory. Oxytocin is also important for healthy psychological attachment to the primary caregiver. It's produced by the hypothalamus and is excreted by the pituitary gland. Most of the early research on this NT is on breastfeeding and attachment.

When were engaged in empathy, as we'll see in Part III, oxytocin is involved. Any time we're building trust, staring into another's eyes, we're getting some oxytocin secreted into our bloodstream, going wherever it needs to go in the body.

Speaking of addiction, oxytocin is connected to serotonin and dopamine. This is a triple-threat cocktail of good happy feelings. This is an excellent reason to get three safe, non-sexual hugs per day. We make eye contact, connect with a human, and maybe share a smile. It's a prescription for feeling good.

Integration Practice: Let your hand guide itself.

Get a pencil and a piece of plain, unlined paper and some lined notebook paper. The first is for drawing with your eyes closed. The lined paper is for you to write down what you're going to think about with your eyes closed. You'll need something legit to cover your eyes too. No cheating.

Make a list of the following situations from your life. You only need to jot down enough words to recall the mood, tone, and feeling clearly. First, remember a stressful situation. Once you have one in mind, mentally consider the following line of self-inquiry. Where did you feel it in your body? What are the other sensations and memories that you recall?

Set your phone timer for 1-2 minutes. Pick up the pencil, and put it at the bottom right corner if you're an analytical person. If you're a dreamer, place the tip at the top left corner. Close your eyes and let your hand move where it naturally wants to draw. Don't help your hand. Rather than draw lines of an object, think instead of the spaces between the line. Let the hand draw the lines, don't guide the hand; the hand is the guide. Let go of the need to drive it. Let it flow.

For extra credit, try the practice without lifting your pencil off the paper for the whole time, and keep it moving.

After the timer goes off, do the same thing with two more experiences. Recall an episode or time of extreme attachment or addiction. Remember, the details aren't going on the paper, just a couple of words. The last scenario to recall is one of profound calm. Do the entire cycle with the most peaceful moment you can think of, create, or remember. If you're not a dreamer, let yourself dream a little. Let the dream guide you. Ask your guides for help. What do you think they're there for?

You don't have to run anymore. They're not coming for you. There is no bullet to try and outrun except the one we shoot ourselves in the foot with when we forget to love ourselves. This practice does a bunch of different things. One significant feature of all these skills we're working on is that you learn that it's possible to let go of the need to push ahead as if you're being shot at. Because you're not being shot at, be present. Relax and observe. Listen to your body. Let it tell you what you need to know.

Do this practice in other ways. Use paint or other color mediums. Any will be fine. What do you like? Choose different experiences. See how you feel. Let the energy stored in your body from toxic stress and trauma move through the hand. It's like dancing your neurons into happiness with your eyes closed from different angles.

What should you do with the drawings that you did with the opposite side of the brain, in a felt-sense, non-intellectual way? I have no idea. You decide. OK, I have one idea, pick which one you'd send as a Christmas card to your ex.

In this chapter, we learned that neurotransmitters could make us run, get to safety, bump up the ole' mood-a-rooney or drop our ass down a spiral. Some increase feelings of well-being with activities that boost dopamine and serotonin and clear out the catecholamines from our system. At the same time, past and current toxic stress blast the stress hormones and NTs that put us into fight mode, even when there's no one attacking us.

Let's be clear; these are simplifications. These neurotransmitters work in many ways in different systems throughout the brain network.

The literature on these aspects of neuroscience is vast. But the purpose of this section was to break it down enough to give the foundation we need to discuss the next topic, your brain.

We haven't not been talking about the brain this whole time. But let's take a look at the brain parts involved in the transmission of neurotransmitters into circuitries that fire every second of our lives without us knowing a damn thing about them. Well, that's all in the past now.

You can have an informed conversation on any one of these topics in the time it takes to walk to the elevator. It's important to acknowledge the value of taking the time to study. Now you know something that perhaps you didn't know. Let's look at the brain parts relevant to our discussion as we continue to focus and clarify how it all fits into the story of your brain on toxic stress and addiction.

Notes

Chapter 9
Your Brain

"Just the facts, ma'am."
-Joe Friday [61]

There are conflicting views in the literature on the precise wiring of the brain. Because the research isn't conclusive and definitive, nor is it "proof" of something, this organization of thought is a particular framework, not to be confused with the standard, textbook, or other anatomical references. Since we don't need everything in the known universe to make a point, it makes sense to save time and learn what we need to know to get done what needs to be done. And what do we need? Well, healing, of course.

Therefore, in keeping with our super-simplified, what-you-need-to-know discussion, what follows are some bare-bones essentials that are required to understand what is happening with us as we experience toxic stress, trauma, and addiction over time. Again, just get a feeling for what's going on. Don't sweat the technical stuff.

---

[61] played by Jack Webb, in the TV show Dragnet (1951-59)

The first thing we need is an overview of the sections of the brain. [62] We have a forebrain,

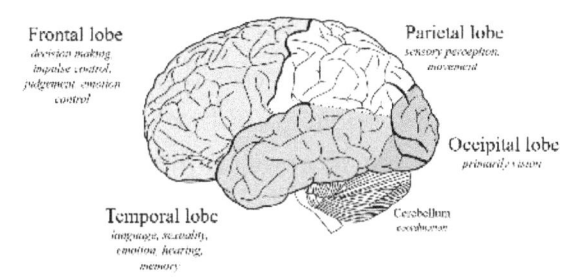

Frontal lobe
*decision making,
impulse control,
judgement, emotion
control*

Parietal lobe
*sensory perception,
movement*

Occipital lobe
primarily vision

Temporal lobe
*language, sexuality,
emotion, hearing,
memory*

Cerebellum
coordination

midbrain, and hindbrain. The largest part of the brain, the cerebrum, is covered by the cerebral cortex.

Forebrain

The forebrain is covered by the cerebral cortex, a gray, wrinkly layer of nerve cells. The largest part of the cerebral cortex is the neocortex, responsible for essential functions such as thinking and doing. The neocortex is divided into four sections or lobes: the frontal, parietal, occipital lobe, and temporal lobes. Each lobe is responsible for batches of processes.

---

62 A more detailed explanation is outside our scope and frankly, not hyper critical to our discussion. Hopefully, you're discussing this with others in your recovery circle as well. It applies to most of us.

Frontal Lobe

The frontal lobe is where all the thinking goes on or is supposed to! Behind the forehead, our frontal lobe reasons, organizes, solves problems, keeps us from taking all our clothes off and running down the street, regulates behavior, memory, and emotions. It makes plans, controls how our face shows emotion, and controls movements. Also, if you're like me and lacking in some of the more refined social skills, this is the area where they'd typically be found. The Prefrontal Cortex is the front most part of the frontal lobe at the forebrain. It's just behind your forehead.

Parietal Lobe

The parietal lobe, located in the upper back area of the brain, is the command and control for seeing, the sense of touch, overall body awareness, and how we perceive spaces and orient ourselves to them. As a control center, this lobe integrates sensory input from all over the body. It also retains our knowledge of the relationships between numbers and how we move objects through space. Here, we comprehend the yoga teacher's instruction, put ourselves in a pose, develop deeper awareness and insights, and balance between left and right.

Temporal Lobe

This lobe is fortunately located near the ears. It's responsible for our ability to hear the teacher over the chatter of girls behind us, separate all of the sensory information, remember what was said and seen, and then produce a way of speaking about the experience. When you use your inner Google to search for just the right word to say to the cutie next to you or an autobiographical memory to share, it's in the temporal lobe that your Google will seek that information.

Occipital Lobe

The occipital lobe is responsible for visual and spatial processing and analysis, and memory of visual information. It funnels the raw sensory input into the perception that can read nonverbal cues in body language.

Midbrain

The midbrain is at the center of your brain. It's the smallest region, essential to us because it contains the largest amount of dopamine-producing neurons. As a connector between our auditory and visual circuitries, the midbrain also controls our body's ability to move; the midbrain is home to our limbic system, composed of the thalamus, hypothalamus, amygdala, and hippocampus. Some researchers include the basal ganglia and cingulate gyrus. We'll consider that an outside issue as the grouping doesn't affect what we're doing here.

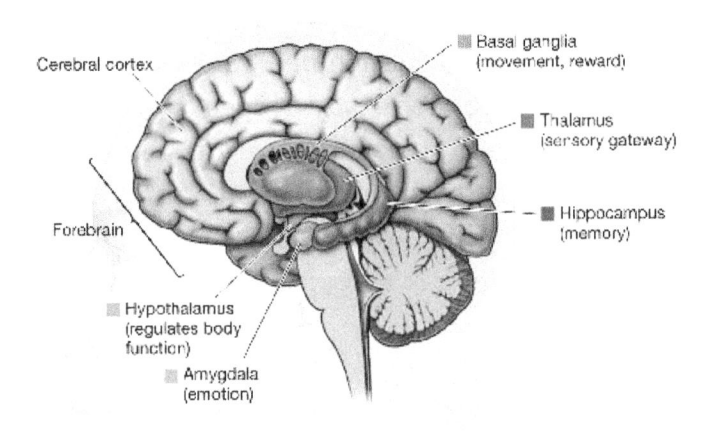

- Cerebral cortex
- Forebrain
- Basal ganglia (movement, reward)
- Thalamus (sensory gateway)
- Hippocampus (memory)
- Hypothalamus (regulates body function)
- Amygdala (emotion)

We need to know about the midbrain because this is where, in the limbic system, the brain processes emotions. It's also where the traumatic results of ACEs live. As we'll discuss further on, healing methods that target the limbic system are key to healing trauma.

Limbic System

The limbic system lives deep in our cerebrum. It is our primitive and ancient survival brain. Cognition, or the ability to think, occurs in the prefrontal cortex, not the limbic. Cognition is the advance of Homo Sapiens[63] over our predecessors.

---

63 "Homo sapiens – the species sapiens (wise) of the genus Homo (man)." Yuval Noah Harari. "Sapiens: A Brief History of Humankind."

Over 70,000 years ago, for some unknown reason, the Cognitive Revolution happened. We created language used to make up stories and create social systems. Yes, it's true; the first thing we did when our brains got big enough was learn how to spread fake news. Fiction, however, is the basis of pretty much every story in our lives that we take as real.

But the limbic, where we feel the feels—our emotional humanity—is also found in fish, amphibians, reptiles, and mammals.

The system perceives and responds to danger, feels safe, and perceives the world. The limbic system provides automatic reactions and shapes our disposition towards the world. That means our tendencies to act, think, and feel distinguish us from others. This is the seat of our sense of ourselves. The ways we look at and respond to the world happen here. Critical to our discussion is that most of our stored trauma lives in the limbic system. We'll address that coming up in more detail.

It's key for us to understand that our temperament can be optimistic and social or short-tempered and irritable. We might be analytical and quiet or relaxed and peaceful. All of this is based on the functioning of our limbic system, which is developed in childhood. This is the seat of our deepest experiences. ACEs are deep experiences. We need deep and powerful healing experiences to heal this stuff. Are you starting to see what this is all about? We make new experiences to rewire the old, toxic experiences. These principles and practices in this book are aimed at healing on a collaborative, universal basis that anyone can learn and embody. It wouldn't be compassionate if it left anyone out. Here are three things that you need to know about your limbic system.

If you have ACEs, your threat perception system is enhanced. You see things as dangerous that other people don't have issues with. Your fear-based survival system is often on high alert when there are no visible threats.

Second, your ability to discern reality from fiction is decreased. Your filter that usually helps distinguish what is relevant and important from what is trivial is broken. You tend to make mountains out of mole hills. It's easy for you to get caught up in irrelevant details that others easily dismiss.

Here's a super important point, especially for people who feel they have an attention deficit. This kind of dysregulation takes us out of the ability to be present at the moment. We're in perpetual distraction, making it difficult for us to engage in normal, everyday situations and interactions. Our compassion and mindful practices help us heal this.

Third, your sense of self is fuzzy and unclear. You may feel the anguish and tension of past experiences in your body. You feel differently than others who are in the same room or party. Your insides don't match their outsides. To avoid or change these feelings, you've developed attachments and addictions to take the edge off.

Is this hitting home at all? Take a moment to discuss or write some feelings down in the Notes section of this chapter.

Thalamus

The thalamus is responsible for the interpretation of sights and sounds. One of its primary functions is to send that sensory data to the cerebral cortex for further analysis.

Hypothalamus

The hypothalamus's primary function is to regulate the pituitary gland and body temperature and sleep. It releases hormones and regulates sexual and other appetites and your feelings about them.

Pituitary Gland

Before we talk about this, please say the word pituitary in a James Earl Jones voice. Try it on friends and family. Look up from the dinner conversation and say, "I feel it in my pituitary," with a very serious look and that commanding presence that you're famous for.

Back to our regularly scheduled programming. The pituitary is a tiny pea behind the center of your skull that connects your nervous system with your endocrine system. The result is hormones that help you grow, metabolize, develop sexually, and reproduce. The pituitary is hard wired to the hypothalamus.

Amygdala

The amygdala is commonly referred to as our inner fire alarm. The fear system comprises the amygdala, the periaqueductal grey, and the hypothalamus. If you've heard about your amygdala, it's because this system is one of the most highly researched areas of brain science. It is a primary focus of current trauma research and the classifications of toxic stress-related disorders.

The amygdala is our threat response survival center. It acts as the central processing unit for sensory input. Because it's connected to the hippocampus, the amygdala is linked to *emotional memories*. This complex area houses a ton of opiate receptor sites associated with our most primal feeling of fear, rage, and that I-need-to-get-me-some-right-now feeling. You know, when the baby-making playlist comes on.[64] Don't hate the amygdala; hate the game. Instead, let's rewrite that narrative to something more compassionate. Love your amygdala but put a leash on it!

Hippocampus

This area is not related to hippopotamuses, but it is related to sea horses. You might notice a slight

---

[64] You could be like, "Baby, your amygdala is fire right now." Let me know how it works out.

resemblance if you took your hippocampus out and put it up next to one of those little guys swimming around in an aquarium. This area is related to forming and organizing memories related to our emotional universe and sense of self. The healthy hippocampus also connects the five senses to these emotional memories. For example, a trigger might give you a feeling that isn't related to anything other than a smell. You smell cologne and realize there's no one nearby, but that song is playing again—the one from that bad experience.

Basal Ganglia

The basal ganglia are neuronal structures deep in the brain's center that connect to the frontal lobes. They're primarily responsible for movement and motor control. Still, the basal ganglia's importance to our addiction and recovery plays a significant role in executive functions, emotional behavior, or how we act out our feelings, reward functions, habits, and addictions. It is also connected to our limbic system.

Extended Amygdala

The extended amygdala is in the center of the amygdala, but it also connects to other areas such as the basal ganglia. It's responsible in part for recognizing rewards. Because it's part of the reward system, it plays a role in the cycle of addiction and its long-term effects.

Periaqueductal gray

The "PAG" is a mass of gray matter that you can find if you poke around in the midbrain. It's thought to be an interface between the forebrain and the brain stem, which is responsible for regulating vital life functions such as breathing, heartbeat, and blood pressure.

When we think deeply about how we feel deeply, it's just a PAG thang. Other functions include cardiovascular, fine motor, pain response, and respiration. Isn't that fascinating?

This simple overview is what we need to look specifically at what happens in your brain on addiction.

Notes

Chapter 10
Your Brain on Addiction

"The greatest impact on morbidity of ACES is in the area of substance abuse and mental health."
-Dr. Robert Anda[65]

Now that we understand a little about the normal function of different parts of the brain, we have a foundation to discuss the effects of addiction on the brain. If you've never really studied this explanation, take a close look. There are some exciting and terrible things going on with us when we engage in the process of serious addiction. However, these same systems can be put to good use in recovery. With proper understanding, practice, and support, we repurpose our circuits back to what they're supposed to do, even better when infused with compassion.

There are three areas of the brain to talk about regarding current addiction research. The dysregulation or disruption of these areas does three things. First, the disruption causes a disruption that creates a disruption that continues. Second,

---
65 samhsa.gov 2012

addiction dulls our ability to feel pleasure and, at the same time, become hypersensitive to stress. We talked about the stress systems earlier, as you'll recall. Think about that for a moment. How sensitive are you to stress? How much real joy and pleasure do you have in life? How have these changed over time in relation to your attachments and addictions? What about in recovery?

The third dysregulation is a loss of function in our executive system or circuitry. It means we don't think clearly or make good emotional decisions. There's difficulty in processing emotions, and our impulse control goes out the window, which causes our impulse control to go out the window. All these neuroadaptations get worse over time without intervention[66].

The simplified big picture of our addiction cycle is that we start with feeling compelled to change due to internal or external triggers. When we respond to such stressful feelings with addictive behavior, we train our brains to get more addicted. This is incentive salience.

If you've been to treatment in the last twenty years, you've probably had a lecture that you forgot

---

66 Substance Abuse and Mental Health Services Administration (US); Office of the Surgeon General (US). Facing Addiction in America: The Surgeon General's Report on Alcohol, Drugs, and Health [Internet]. Washington (DC): US Department of Health and Human Services; 2016 Nov. PMID: 28252892.

or a pamphlet you lost on this topic. But understanding incentive salience is key to unlocking the mystery of why we just can't stop and, more importantly, why we need to stop completely to begin healing. What does incentive salience mean?

The incentive or the action you take associated with the high becomes part of the high. It's salient because the goal or reward is clear or feels within reach, even though we can be many steps away from getting the high we seek. The ritual of planning, seeking, and acquiring our addictive thing is part of the high. It reinforces the high by strengthening the cognition that you can change it when you have an uncomfortable feeling. All the planning, seeking, and acquiring is as much a part of the addiction, at a dopamine reward level, as the drug itself.

You know that feeling when your mouth is getting dry, and you're not even getting high? Because usually, in the words of the legendary George Thorogood, when your mouth is getting dry, you're pretty high. When the impulse decision to reach out to your cocaine dealer makes you pass wet gas, which you find enjoyable. These experiences that are associated with addiction become part of the cycle that keeps us addicted. But they do something more insidious. With every loop down the spiral of active participation in our addiction, the rut carved by addiction into our grey matter takes us deeper and deeper until we stop, or it stops us.

We all have our bottoms or places where we decide we've sunk low enough and have realized that it's time to rebuild. That decision can be made at any place on the attachment spectrum. Utilize the principle, not the detail.

To enter recovery, stay out of the funnel and thrive on the road to self-mastery, we need to understand the realities that we're dealing with. Most people don't make it to recovery. Serious addicts have low chances of survival. Of those that do find recovery, most don't stay. According to the Surgeon General, "More than 60 percent of people treated for a substance use disorder experience relapse within the first year after they are discharged from treatment, and a person can remain at increased risk of relapse for many years." This is borne out in my experience over quite a few years. Compassionate Recovery attempts to identify, address and heal many of these whys that keep us from peace and happiness.

The work you're doing right now will help keep you out of the funnel. Keep going. Talk to people about it. Get support and stay in touch with them. Be honest, be consistent.

The Cycle of Addiction

Pre-occupation/Planning Stage:
Prefrontal Cortex

Addiction takes over our forebrain's Stop and Go systems. The latter drives us to seek pleasure (attachment) or avoid suffering (aversion). The more incentive salience and subsequent addictive reinforcement that sinks in, the deeper the cycle burns new neurological wiring that is addiction. It gets burned in, then re-burned constantly over time. Because of this, addiction becomes an addiction. It's like holding a mirror up to a mirror. As our neurons cascade, so does our ability to Stop.

The more you use, the more you need to use until your entire life becomes about the drug. There is nothing else. No children. No community. No plan for tomorrow. This example makes the process clear enough for our purposes. Not all drugs act the same way, and there are many factors involved in different types of addictions. But you don't have to go way down the rabbit hole to be addicted or to be in recovery. We stop when we're ready to stop. Hopefully, that's before we die.

Here's what you need to know. You can use your Go system to travel in the direction you want to go. Repurpose your organic internal systems. Compassionate Recovery can be your dilithium crystals to recharge and rewire the main core of your central processing system so you can get that starship out to some new and better galaxies.

When your Go system is working, your ability to make plans and decisions toward goals is fine. But the Go system gets hijacked by addiction, which becomes the only goal on which all decisions must be focused. That's because incentive salience kicks in glutamate, another excitatory neurotransmitter. We're triggered by cues that increase activity in the prefrontal cortex, increasing incentive salience. Some would call this obsessive thinking. Is the point becoming salient?

Cues stimulate us to seek. The seeking itself becomes its own reinforcing cue, and the whole system of serious attachment or addiction becomes a self-perpetuating sinkhole. That's why we can't stop just a little. Cutting back doesn't work. Any amount of the addictive behavior can and does create the entire chemical cascade all over again. Control of the addiction is an illusion. [67] Total abstinence from addiction is the only way to unlearn and re-burn the new programmable memory that we need.

---

[67] A very stupid illusion at that, once you see how it works. There's no way to control it, unless you can adjust your brain at the molecular level through sheer concentration, in which case I should be reading your book.

We go when we don't need to go, and we struggle to stop when we need to stop. As you may have guessed, the Stop system is supposed to inhibit the Go circuitry. In addition to being the control center for stress and emotion, the Stop system controls habitual responses and can inhibit incentive salience. Because of that fact, you can recover.

It may sound like a lot to absorb, but it's better to know what's coming so we can learn how to cope with life as it presents itself to us, rather than fantasize about it. Slow down the Go and ramp up the Stop, and you've got yourself a new automatic response to triggers, cues, and those nasty funnel traps.

All of this happens automatically. In the automatic systems, we learned about earlier, the effects of addiction—dysregulation—and subsequent neuroadaptations occur. That's why we focus our medicine on areas where we can build new, self-compassion circuits. Maybe it's counter-adapting the neuroadaptation. We bring the deep healing to the deep places that words can't access. We know what we're doing and why, which empowers our practice of recovery.

In the compassionate view, however, treatments that seek to reduce harm rather than demand total abstinence are still helpful and not seen as unfavorable. We all work with the capacity and understanding available to us. Understanding this about ourselves and each other is the pre-frontal cortex and compassion at work.

Neuroadaptations from Addiction

The consequences of addiction are changes to how we feel, think and act. This part of the brain is responsible for organizing our thoughts, planning our days, figuring out where to be and when all the thoughts, plans, and calculations are about the addiction. The good news is that we can form new thoughts in recovery, leading to new feelings that can become our baseline instead of hypo or hyperarousal.

Addiction causes impairments to the regular operation of the forebrain, affecting all the areas of our common humanity that we discussed at the beginning. The solutions must also be applied to our mental, emotional, physical, and spiritual dimensions. As our addictions progress, we lose the ability to think and act correctly, and we get impulse control disorders. We show little or no self-control, are irritable or numb, and can't solve the problem of our life. That stress can push us right back into the cycle.

The prefrontal cortex in the planning stage interacts with the basal ganglia and extended amygdala during the binge\intoxication and withdrawal\negative affect stages. These three systems get out of balance in addiction, making going into addiction easier than stopping ourselves from the impulse.

Binge/Intoxication Stage: Basal Ganglia

The binge or intoxication stage is party time, baby! Let's get down. Come on! Drink up, smoke up, shoot up, eat up, sex it up and keep it up. That's how we do. Why? Because the basal ganglia controls the rewards and pleasurable effects of our addictions and the development of powerful habits that become compulsive addictions.

The Basal Ganglia connects different brain regions. It reaches into several brain lobes with two main branches, the reward branch of circuits and the habit branch of circuits. We care about the reward circuitry, where we get a nice dopamine and opioid combo hit from engagement with our addiction. Incentive salience activities, as we learned, make the seeking ritual a juicy reward activity by blasting the excitatory and pleasurable neurotransmitters long before we get to the dope man's house, let alone feel the rush of the needle. This system is where the addiction digs into our brains like a burrowing dung beetle. All the things that stimulate us, cue us, or that we associate with the reward become part of craving and seeking and using our addictive stuff of choice.

The other branch of the basal ganglia is the habit circuit. Because of the dopamine reward and the excitement from glutamates, dynorphins and endorphins create changes in the circuitries that increase our seeking behaviors to become compulsive. These can be habits, but as we know, a mere habit would be a welcome change from our serious addictions.

The two things that create the binge/intoxication experience are the intense, obsessive craving and a compulsion to get that dope, whatever our dope is.

Neuroadaptations from Addiction

The neuroadaptations in the basal ganglia due to addiction can drastically reduce our ability to feel pleasure in everyday life. Like depression, we lost interest in tasty food, good friends, and even good sex. Over time, the addictive substance or activity feels less potent because our circuits adapt. Because of this, the dope is the only thing that makes us feel better and is, therefore, all we want. And the more we use, the more harm we cause ourselves. Self-compassion is getting clean and sober. Don't you think? You're worth it. Get started today.

Withdrawal/Negative Affect Stage: Extended Amygdala

What goes up must come down. And so it goes for those on the spectrum of addiction. After a point in our binge cycle, the party ends. Everybody went home hours ago. There you sit, unable or unwilling to figure out your next move.

The physical and emotional reactions in the withdrawal stage vary depending on the specific addiction and the individual. Whatever your dope is, you know all about the kind of hangovers that you experience. Be careful not to stake a claim as some sort of real addict that knows withdrawal-like no one else. Whether you wake up dehydrated and gagging on your knees with your face against the crust of last night's vomit from too much $2 Tuesday Tacos and beers, or fall to the ground shaking and sobbing outside of a bagel place due to excruciating withdrawal from a toxic narcissist, suffering is suffering. Yet, for us, this is not the end of the cycle; far from it.

We get back on the wild bull and ride it until we wake up shattered and broken. That sucks, so better get on out and grab some more hair of the steer that bit you. And so it goes. We all have our version of the story.[68]

We've all been there, and sadly, many of us will never get out of the deadly loop of addiction. You don't have to be one of them. It's not necessary to prove that you're more of an addict or less of an addict. We are all on different spectrums with various issues, physical, mental, emotional, and

---

68 Try writing yours out.

spiritual. To practice compassion is to know we're all in our own cycles of suffering. Lend a hand. Be kind.

The extended amygdala, as we know, is integral to the process of stress. During withdrawal, it's the center of our anxiety and general crankiness. In the withdrawal/negative affect stage, the reward systems we learned about get less rewarding. The stress neurotransmitters dynorphin and CRF start blasting through the extended amygdala. There's no way to feel OK in this kind of stress NT cascade with the simultaneous lack of dopamine. Here's what you need to know.

When we're in this negative feeling state, we are compelled to pick up our addiction again regardless of what aspect of our humanity it manifests on. If you recall, we teach our brains that we must have the addictive thing. This is part of the education of destruction that happens in our addict brains. Until now, because now we know about it and can start working on the healing. That's what this is about.

Neuroadaptations from Addiction

The cycle again burns itself into our neurology, setting our NTs into constantly firing stress into our bodies. We feel and act like we're in withdrawal more and more, even when we're engaging in our addiction. The adaptation, however, is that this situation keeps working this way even when we get sober. That's why it's a neuroadaptation. If you're not an addict but have had a hangover, imagine feeling that way most of the time, at least on an emotional level.

The other aspect of neuroadaptation that sticks with us from the withdrawal cycle repetition over time is sensitivity to the object of our addiction. This is what you need to know. Over time, due to what happens in the extended amygdala as we pound ourselves with addiction is that the addiction doesn't get us off anymore. It's more of temporary relief from the suffering of physical, mental, and emotional withdrawal. Then there's the spiritual black hole, but we'll get to that later.

Additional Neuroadaptations in the Limbic System

There is some crossover between the neuroadaptations of addiction and those of trauma. In addition to the inability to respond to regular pleasure, the amygdala, as our alarm system, can fire at the wrong time and be deadened when we need to know there is risk ahead. It's like going backward and forwards internally at the same time. We can also get a hair trigger to a pent-up inner rage, which leads to violence. If we're on the hyperarousal swing of our window of tolerance, we'll have ramped up fears and anxieties.

Conversely, if we're in the hypo or low end, we're likely to find ourselves couch-locked with a bag of Doritos in one hand and a 2-liter of Diet Coke in the other. If that's not wacky enough, dysregulation in the limbic can also lead to hypersexuality and reduced inhibition. No joke here; it can create a disorder that causes the insertion of inappropriate objects in the mouth.[69]

Our appetite can get disordered, leading to binge eating, emotional eating, and other disorders on top of the addiction that caused it. Memories, which are already foggy from not being present in our bodies with our full hearts and minds, get worse in short- and long-term memory. If we didn't already have a learning disorder from ACEs, that could become impaired as other disorders of cognition, including Alzheimer's. The same damage we cause to our hippocampus is the same as what causes this deterioration of memory that we may recognize in older people. It can happen sooner if we fry our limbic too badly.

In summary, the takeaways are clear. The more addicted we get, the more addicted we get. The more addicted we become, the less our brains can experience pleasure due to dopamine hijacking. Even after we sober up, this problem typically continues. It may or may not be reversible.

We can, however, make positive and healing changes with our Compassionate Recovery principles and practices. The practices affect the parts of the brain that are affected by ACEs and

---

69 Hyperorality https://www.ncbi.nlm.nih.gov/medgen/325386

addiction. We take a bottom-up approach rather than a top-down one.

The top-down is working from the forebrain through talk therapy. At the same time, bottom-up focuses on the limbic system through physical disciplines such as high-intensity interval training, yoga, and martial arts. Would bowling count in that? Good question. Wherever you get your zen on is good.

The toxic stress that contributed to setting you up for addiction also helps keep you addicted and on the downward spiral mentally, emotionally, physically, and spiritually. Let's take a closer look at your brain on trauma and the setup for addiction.

Notes

Chapter 11
Your Brain on Trauma

"The dysregulation may be present before the person takes a drug, or it may be caused by constant (chronic) drug-taking or induced by a psychosocial stressor, such as trauma. Or it could be all three.[70]"
- Carlton K. Erickson

One of the main problems for trauma victims is ignorance in the clinical field. Bessel Van der Kolk, MD, and his colleagues have worked to bring the research findings on trauma to the forefront of clinical knowledge. The hard truth is that, due to political and financial issues, the truth about trauma has been swept under the rug for decades while victims suffered. In the past 15-20 years, research funding into trauma has opened up again. But the front-line treatment providers are still catching up to bring healing solutions to those of us who need them.

There are three ways to survive trauma, and there aren't clear lines between them. The first and most

---

[70] The Science of Addiction: From Neurobiology to Treatment (Norton Professional Books)

common is that most of us wind up in a posttraumatic decline, living a life of severely impaired mental and medical health. You see us on the street before we become victims of homicide or suicide.

If we're more fortunate, we might wind up with a life chronically disturbed by events of a posttraumatic nature. These may or may not be in response to normal life circumstances. They may happen from unknown triggers. We get hijacked by past trauma. It interrupts our lives, but at least we still have lives.

The other survival mode is the one you're on, luckily, the path of recovery. Everything we're doing in this book, the path of Compassionate Recovery, is about this. We learn to not only overcome the past but to live a healthy and satisfying life of a compassionate community, conscious connection, and meaningful work. We don't have to do it alone. There's a whole world of hurt out there that needs us. This work is vital to them. Remember that. You are important to someone you're going to help in the future.

Trauma is not an incident. Trauma is a response. Our brain circuitries and systems respond to intense, toxic stress that we cannot escape from nor cope with. It can be short, episodic stress or the long-term, chronic variety. We began the story of Compassionate Recovery with the story ACEs, which is the story of trauma. We covered the effects of

ACEs as they related to us and focused our understanding on the dysregulation that occurs in our brains due to the trauma of addiction.

Addiction is, for most of us, a response to ACEs. Not everyone who is traumatized gets addicted, and not every addict has ACEs. But the relationship is higher than would occur by chance alone. Addiction is the most common of all adverse health effects caused by ACEs.

In this chapter, we'll add important knowledge on the brain dysregulations and subsequent neuroadaptations that happen as our brains develop in childhood, which precede addiction.

This material continues to be difficult on several levels. Remember, even if this work is uncomfortable or difficult to process, it will enhance the vital self-empowerment of your healing. You're doing great!

As you may have guessed, our stress regulation system isn't so regulated. The neuroadaptations that happen are often stress-related disorders. If we don't have one of those, we can still experience problems such as responding to stress when there is no stressful event happening at that moment. Our amygdala, the alert system, becomes overactive. We swing out of our window of tolerance into anxiety and avoidance of stressors. We can be jumpy and uncertain to the point of hypervigilance.

Since the hippocampus becomes undersized, which is strongly supported in the trauma literature, we lose memory and the ability to calm ourselves down. We can be plagued with ongoing confusion in everyday situations and be disoriented, have obsessive thoughts, nightmares, and sleep difficulty. Flashbacks can be of some trivial detail of a traumatic incident or manifest as a feeling of unease, panic, or sickness. The hippocampus typically has a stress-reducing effect on the amygdala, but this also becomes impaired. When this part of the brain doesn't respond correctly to danger signals, it's hard to keep ourselves safe.

Because our thalamus is affected, we can also have difficulty processing sights and sounds. Our prefrontal cortex, as in addiction, becomes impaired to the point where we have all sorts of behavioral, emotional, and learning problems.

In non-stressful times, it's still hard for us to think clearly, make plans, troubleshoot, problem-solve, and control our impulses. In stress, these are all exacerbated. Toxic stress burns into our neuronal structures, creating layers of dysregulation as our young brains develop.

Concentrated levels of catecholamine released during a stress response immediately impair the top-down functioning of the prefrontal cortex. At the same time, the intense emotionality of the reward system and habit formation is on full blast, so we are learning beneath the surface to be more traumatized as time goes on. Many of us become addicted to this very process of high stress and intense emotions[71]. That may be a setup for trauma-bond relationships where the victim stays willingly with their abuser.

Healthy Release

In the wild, when an animal is traumatized by an attack from a predator but not seriously wounded, it will automatically do a healthy release of the trauma by shaking violently until the neurotransmitter circuits reset. If they're trapped and suffering, and it's prolonged, healthy release can't happen.

Of all the 9/11 first responders on the ground in the burning devastation, those who received immediate trauma release recovered without incurring later symptoms of stress-related disorders. Dr. Tian Dayton worked in New York in 2011 as an on-scene therapist, where she employed a type of psychodrama role play. In this approach, roles are acted out, seats are switched, and intense emotions are given a voice before they get buried. When we rapidly acknowledge and release trauma, we can be free of it. This is a self-care skill that can be acquired.

---

71 Amy F.T. Arnsten, Murray A. Raskind, Fletcher B. Taylor, Daniel F. Connor,

The effects of stress exposure on prefrontal cortex: Translating basic research into successful treatments for post-traumatic stress disorder, Neurobiology of Stress, Volume 1,2015, Pages 89-99, ISSN 2352-2895, https://doi.org/10.1016/j.ynstr.2014.10.002

Role-playing techniques are effective methods for integrating parts of ourselves. The methods can be instrumental in recovery.

True, the first responders she treated on-site were adults who had plenty of support and were doing something heroic. They weren't kids being abused beyond comprehension over time. Trauma in adulthood is also damaging but is not in the same developmental time frame. There's more brain development to cope and recover in the adult brain. Growing up with trauma is more difficult to heal.

Any trauma that is left unresolved, unacknowledged, and unexpressed becomes a problem. When we're traumatized in the womb by our mother's alcoholism or in early childhood by a father that molests us, we don't even have words to express it. Our brains adapt to the suffering. Many who've suffered have not received the treatment that could have helped us, but those days are over.

You need to know that if you internalize the ideas in this book and practice consistently with the tools presented here, you are going to heal.

You are not your trauma. You are not your addiction. These are experiences. You are a whole being that is much bigger than these experiences.

Breathe in. Breathe out.

These are just ripples on the surface of an infinite sea of consciousness. Own your vastness.

According to the National Institutes of Health, *"7.7 million adults have co-occurring mental and substance use disorders. This doesn't mean that one caused the other and it can be difficult to determine which came first.*

Of the 20.3 million adults with substance use disorders, 37.9% also had mental illnesses.

Among the 42.1 million adults with mental illness, 18.2% also had substance use disorders."[72]

If you tell someone—in or out of recovery that you have a trauma-related disorder—most people use PTSD as a blanket term—they're going to say, "Me, too." It's more commonly talked about than it used to be in recovery, but that doesn't mean enough is being done about it. That changes now.

This section will dial in our terms, clear up some misconceptions, and review past and present clinical perspectives on trauma-related disorders. Again, it's not comprehensive and is simplified for clarity based on what we need to know to be informed about healing ourselves and our communities.

With the advent of fMRI advanced brain imaging technology[73] in the early 1990s, enormous gains have

---

72 https://nida.nih.gov/drug-topics/trends-statistics/infographics/comorbidity-substance-use-other-mental-disorders

73 functional magnetic resonance imaging (fMRI)

been made in brain science. Most of what we've covered so far is because of this shift. One result is that we know more about the diagnostic criteria for what ails, so many of us are catching up to our long-neglected realities. I say long neglected because our school and legal systems, recovery programs, and most of our families have not understood us.

We in the addiction spectrum have been punished for being punished. For example, learning disabilities due to emotional blunting and hypertoxic stress cause behavioral problems that get us in trouble. As we develop, the problems compound.

The first healing that we need is self-compassion. We study ourselves with compassion and try to understand that we are who we are for many reasons, some of which are not in our control. However, our healing and self-empowerment are in no one else's control but our own.

The understanding of traumatic response syndromes is advanced enough now that new diagnostic criteria are replacing older models. These are targeted towered interventions among children, as screening for ACEs has improved over the decades. Dr. Nadine-Burke Harris, former Surgeon General of California, implemented ACE screenings in her pediatric clinic as a matter of protocol.

There are many volumes written in this field. Again, we have a brief overview of the essential points so we can be conversant and informed with reliable, evidence-based information. Inaccurate information circulates and often sticks in recovery circles. You're better equipped to help yourself and others when you know facts instead of popular ideas. There's plenty in the footnotes throughout this book if you want to get deeper. Don't rule out online learning and in-person degrees.

There is a lot of work to be done. You will impact many people as an addict. It might as well be one of compassion and healing instead of that stuff we used to do.

We can find many different terms in the literature to name our problems. The current effort in the field is geared toward creating a more informed set of criteria for diagnosing and treating complex traumas that occur over time. We need to know that distinct types of trauma cause various kinds of dysregulations in our lives. Depending on what happens in the child or adult developmental cycle, there are apparent differences in effects and any potential for resiliency.

The earlier trauma happens, the sooner dysregulation in development occurs. Our brains develop in stages that depend largely on one another. When there's an interruption from the pre-natal, infancy, toddler, latency, or age 6 to puberty, adolescence before the adult life cycle, it's happening to a brain in development. An older brain, like yours[74], is developed enough physically, socially, and experienced in terms of finding needed resources. All of these contribute to a more fully formed human's ability to recover faster.

Although children are more vulnerable to stress and trauma than adults, both will be able to recover more easily from Type I than Type II traumas.

Type I Trauma

Type I trauma is the response to a single, shocking, and unexpected incident. Since it occurs without warning, such an unexpected shock to our system is severe. It might be something that's nobody's fault, like an earthquake or car accident. It could also be an intentional act such as abuse, rape, assault, or a larger attack on a community such as a riot or terrorism. Type I trauma also happens when we witness intense and out-of-the-ordinary experiences[75].

Classic PTSD

Before we move on, let me clarify something about labels and diagnoses. When reading about

---

74 But you look fantastic!

75 Courtois, C. A., & Ford, J. D. (Eds.). (2009). Treating complex traumatic stress disorders: An evidence-based guide. The Guilford Press.

trauma, addiction, hearing people's stories, or just reading a new report that brings something up for us, instead of going into a spiral, try this. Rather than look at the lists of symptoms and say, "Yeah, that's me," instead, take a deep breath, read a little and pause to let it sink in. Reflect on the following questions:

How true is this for me?

What feelings does it bring up?

How is the fear part of me responding to this?

What do I genuinely want to feel right now?

How can the principles and practices in Compassionate Recovery help support me?

There is disagreement, even contention, due to political and pharmaceutical interests, among the different agencies that decide things like what mental disorder we get labeled with. You might get diagnosed with something inaccurate by a clinician simply to get you into treatment according to insurance guidelines. The DSM-V, Diagnostic and Statistical Manual, is the most used to diagnose mental disorders. However, it is based not only on research but rather on consensus and lobbying.

There has been significant progress in research since the old days when PTSD, like addiction, was a bad word. The current knowledge base is represented here.

With this in mind, we can consider the older terms and those representing more recent thinking and research. Remember, if you identify with these things, don't over-identify. You are not your disorder.

In the immediate aftermath of a traumatic event, we can experience the following symptoms for a while. However, a PTSD diagnosis usually means we've had them for a month to several years.

The symptoms of Post-Traumatic Stress Disorder are in four categories; intrusive thoughts, avoidance of people, places, and things that trigger, and changes in mood[76] and thought such as negative thoughts about oneself, including horror, intense shame, or total detachment.

Arousal. Think about the window of tolerance and all the triggers out there. Someone with classic PTSD may have arousal problems such as what the Alcoholics Anonymous book called restless, irritable, and discontent. Behaviors can be reckless and destructive to ourselves and others. If that sounds like addiction, you need to know that PTSD, like ACEs, doesn't usually occur in isolation.

I had a neighbor once named John. He was a veteran and had served in the Vietnam war. When we met in the 1990s, he was a drug dealer that loved to give friends like me lines of cocaine, tablespoons of GHB out of a bottle, and all the dirt weed one could ask for. All this took place in front of one of those old-style 60" rear projection screens that showed

---

[76] Extra credit if you can name the areas of the brain for mood and thought or congition.

endless porn on an uncensored satellite from Mexico.

John was cool and generous. He was also a serious addict with bad PTSD. Sometimes we'd be sitting there enjoying the strippers he'd brought home, and he'd suddenly disappear. You'd find him in the hallway, pressed against the wall, a loaded handgun in his hand.

"John, what the fuck? Are you OK?".

"Shhhh. GET DOWN! GET DOWN!" would be his response. He'd snap out of it at some point, and we'd get back to business as usual. I don't know if the strippers even noticed.

My friend had the Type I trauma and the subsequent PTSD that comes from experiencing and participating in the horrors of war. Like so many vets, he treated the confusion and suffering with drugs and alcohol.

That doesn't have to happen anymore.

Type II Trauma

Type II trauma isn't single incident related. It is complex. For that reason and clarity, we'll refer to it as complex trauma. This type of trauma has three characteristics. First, it is repetitive and prolonged. Second, it involves betrayal, abandonment, and harm by primary caregivers. Third, while complex traumas such as domestic violence, community violence, war, genocide, or enslavement can happen in adulthood, the general focus is on the critical periods of childhood development, as we will see. Keep in mind that, according to the literature, children are the most traumatized class of humans on the planet.

Post-traumatic effects have characteristics that are not included in Type I trauma. They occur in the four dimensions of humanity discussed in Chapter 1. First, it involves somatic or physical distress. In the emotional domain, we lose the ability to regulate. Mentally, we disassociate from our experiences. Additionally, we wind up in spiritual distress.

Ongoing, systematic emotional abuse, such as what I experienced in between beatings, cracked my psyche. In these cases, our sense of being is shattered and remains disorganized as we try to grow up. These complex, personal traumas inflicted by people we rely on for our survival put us at higher risk for PTSD, anxiety, and other disorders than Type I traumas.

Because these involve what is considered a fundamental betrayal, complex trauma disrupts our most fundamental needs. Those are physical integrity or control of our physical humanity. Another need affected is the ability to develop a healthy, clear, and organized self-identity. We also need a secure attachment to our caregivers to model quality human interactions based on qualities such as compassion and generosity.

Complex Trauma in the Developmental Cycle

In explaining complex trauma through the cycle of child development, please note that other factors can cause these symptoms. It is, however, quite certain that complex traumas cause them.

Infancy

Without proper soothing, caring, and nurturing by caregivers during the critical developmental stage of infancy, the brain's stress system that we learned about earlier gets hijacked into survival mode. Babies interpret the chaos of sensory stimulation by integrating with their caregiver through mutual eye contact, being held and cleaned, vocal sounds, and facial and other movements by caregivers.

A trusting relationship with caregivers is critical for developing a sense of self at this stage. This stability allows us to learn early physical and emotional self-regulation. When trauma happens instead, the range of problems includes difficulty with nursing, speech, sleep, delays in potty training, excessive wetting, rage, separation anxiety, inability to stop crying, or total withdrawal.

If it goes on and soothing doesn't happen, an infant won't thrive and will become detached from the world and caregivers. The worst cases result in illness and death.

Toddler to Grade School

Normal development in this stage involves developing a basic sense of self-identity, further self-regulation, and the ability to learn and speak a language. If complex trauma, discussed later, occurs, the development of emotional regulation is disrupted, and a disorganized, distressed sense of self emerges. These issues begin to layer onto one another to create physical, socio-emotional, and behavioral problems and regression of functioning back to an earlier stage, such as soiling and wetting. If violence, neglect, and loss continue, the child doesn't develop self-control, a positive outlook, or the ability to trust and feel secure with relationships. Additionally, more severe problems may occur—fears, anxieties, tantrums, depression, encopresis, or involuntary pooping. As a child in this sensitive and critical time, we may feel inadequate and ugly and deserve the abuse. We can be filled with terror, rage, shame, or all the above. But it can be worse.

Trauma bonding in children or adults, known earlier as Stockholm syndrome, happens when we're seduced or groomed into a secret, special relationship. We may get a lot of presents and attention. When combined with sexual stimulation, our normal attachment circuitry[77] is used against us

---

[77] Later we'll discuss in terms of healthy attachment vs. unhealthy attachment-addiction.

as we're trained to be bonded with our perpetrators. We've read about extreme cases when children (and adults) are treated in excessively cruel ways for extended periods. When this happens, we are likely to still cling to the perp for dear life, as they are the ones on whom our very survival depends. Victims can identify with and become loyal to and protective of their perps. This can create a disassociation, a dysregulation that is a key feature that distinguishes ordinary from complex types of trauma. In this split state, we feel loved-hated, appreciated-unworthy, or valued-shamed. This confusion and disorganization of self-value persists.

Adolescence

Our psychological development in these years is about forming our own identity as unique and beautiful beings, able to express love and connect with life in all its complexity. It's about finding value in who we are and who we're becoming. But if the unresolved shadows from our earlier childhood are still blocking our radiance, the usual questioning of ourselves turns into something dark. Where we'd typically hyper-focus on every pimple and new hair, if we come into adolescence with a sense of being a helpless human being, filled with guilt and shame, these get magnified intensely. We might even be among those who walk around feeling filthy, disgusting, stupid, worthless, and permanently broken.

You are not broken.

You are who you are in this moment.

It's not always easy. This moment may suck. However, it is, gently place the hand of self-compassion on your heart. Place the other on your face, belly, or other soft spots. Let it be warm and nurturing. Notice the raw physical aspect of how you feel.

What is the emotional current flowing at this moment? How is it connected to your body? Just notice. What emotional feeling do you need right now? What would it feel like if you received that?

Being, just this moment, compassion's way. Say to yourself, mentally or out loud, whatever that feeling is that you need to feel, say, "May I feel that." Repeat this self-compassion healing mantra over and over softly as many tears as you have cried.

Dedicate this practice to the person that you will help heal. That person will be happy to find you. Bless any new tears of theirs, or yours, to be seeds of compassion on the path.

When the path of becoming an adult is disrupted in our circuits, we must find a release. The shaming and self-blaming for how we feel and for the abuse becomes addiction, self-mutilation, binging-purge, hyper-sexuality, and a high-risk attitude with all the logical behaviors that come with it.

These actions are attempts to cope and self-regulate. They are a way to feel in control of our physical and emotional space that has been or continues to be violated.

Adulthood

As discussed earlier, the adult brain and personality are much better equipped to handle and recover from traumas. But when we consider the challenges that many around our planet are experiencing right now, it will tear open the heart of compassion. According to the trauma literature, there are too many. War, poverty, community violence, political, racial, religious, gender and sexual identity violence, prison, human trafficking and forced prostitution, being held as a sex slave[78], being in a cult or dictatorship, or being a first responder. We can be traumatized for who we are on our common physical, emotional, mental, or spiritual dimensions. It is on all these that we harm each other, so it's on everyone that we need to apply the healing medicine[79].

---

78 unwillingly

79 Courtois, C. A., & Ford, J. D. (2013). Treatment of complex trauma: A sequenced, relationship-based approach. Guilford Press.

Complex PTSD

The classic PTSD definition is overused and fails to capture the impact of chronic, multiple, complex traumas on our little developing brains. Complex PTSD is also caused by interpersonal, inescapable factors in our physical, mental, family, and social universes. Complex PTSD was initially focused on children but is now considered to be appliable in adults, according to the Veteran's Administration.

The National Center for PTSD, Veterans Administration says that,

"During long-term traumas, the victim is generally held in a protracted state of captivity, physically or emotionally. In these situations, the victim is under the control of the perpetrator and unable to get away from the danger. Examples of such traumatic situations include: concentration camps, Prisoner of War camps, prostitution brothels, long-term domestic violence, long-term child physical abuse, long-term child sexual abuse, and organized child exploitation rings.

The ICD-11, or International Classification of Diseases 11th Revision, is a text written by international researchers for WHO, the World Health Organization. It classifies not just mental disorders but all diseases and medical conditions.

The ICD-11 says that Complex PTSD happens after exposure to a series of horrific and threatening events. These are mainly prolonged and repetitive and involve being held captive in some way. If all the requirements for PTSD are met, and we have problems in affect or emotional regulation, terrible beliefs about ourselves as being diminished, defeated, or worthless, as well as feelings of shame, guilt, or failure to stop the abuse, and impairments to our personal, family, social, educational, occupational, and other areas of life, we may have Complex PTSD. If you have questions, seek a medical diagnosis from a qualified professional familiar with this research.

Dissociation is a key issue that separates the complex from classic PTSD. It is splitting or unlinking ourselves from the experience as if it is happening to someone else. This is a normal, universal response to a life-threatening event.[80] If the trauma isn't resolved, such as in healthy release, it can lead to various affective disorders.

We can see that when compared to the diagnosis of Classic PTSD, Complex PTSD covers everything that we're missing to explain our ACEs and addictions. This is the one that applies to most of us. Rather than considering Complex trauma or Complex PTSD as a self-diagnosis, consider this a definition and a guideline for healing.

It has substance abuse under it and other mental health issues. Many of these can be healed significantly by our work with Compassionate

---

80 *Steinberg & Schnall, 2000*

Recovery practices. When we feel sadness and suicidal thoughts, anger issues, dissociation, shame, guilt, distrust, hopelessness, and despair, we can hold space for ourselves and each other. We practice compassion and mindfulness and know suffering is common to everyone. All these things we listed above can be healed with self-compassion and a robust, new script. Call it a Sober Script. It's worth a try, don't you think?

Practice:
Write a New Sober Script

Start a new journal dedicated to what is important to you in recovery. Use those values to write about what your decisions will be like, based on those, rather than impulses and unseen triggers.

Develop the voice of the best sober coach you could ask for. It can even be the voice of a hero or favorite, trusted figure. Start writing with this voice guiding you.

Be your own best healer. Soul travelers like us learn that we can stand on our own two feet, but we are also willing to ask for and follow wise counsel from our Circle of Safety. Talk to them about your Sober Script. Develop the ability to discern what is best for you within your own heart and mind.

Some of us are unable to make decisions for ourselves. Others won't listen to a word from anyone. But to be in full recovery long-term, we need to develop the Wisdom of Compassion. That means we can meditate and reflect deeply, knowing who we are and what's important to us and that it's OK if these values change over time. Remember, we proceed on spirals, not straight lines.

Make notes in your new Sober Script (or whatever you want to name it) journal as you progress in recovery as to the thoughts you'd like to have about yourself, how you would like to feel about your connection to yourself, and to the world. It's up to you, and you will do a better job than anyone else!

This concludes Part II: Trauma, Addiction, and the Brain: What We Need to Know. If you've gone through the chapters in order, which is not necessary but recommended, you have a good sense of the scope of the problems we face. It was challenging material[81] to learn about but absolutely fundamental to a recovery life plan based on compassion and wisdom.

Now let's focus on some healing solutions to all of these things we've learned about.

---

81 If you think this was difficult to read, imagine spending five years researching and writing it with an ACE score of 9. Just sayin'.

Notes

Part III

Healing Your Brain: Compassion Circuitries

Compassion

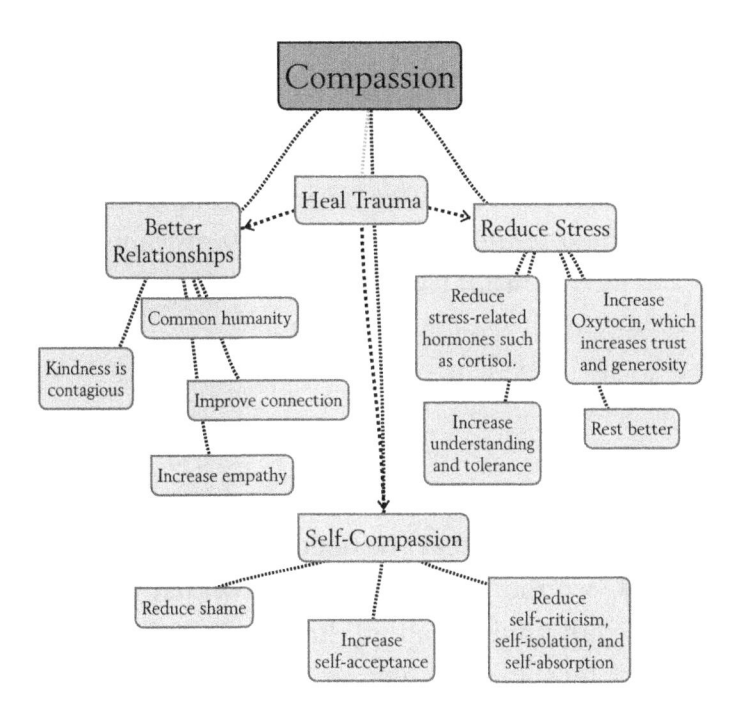

- **Heal Trauma**
- **Better Relationships**
  - Kindness is contagious
  - Common humanity
  - Improve connection
  - Increase empathy
- **Reduce Stress**
  - Reduce stress-related hormones such as cortisol.
  - Increase understanding and tolerance
  - Increase Oxytocin, which increases trust and generosity
  - Rest better
- **Self-Compassion**
  - Reduce shame
  - Increase self-acceptance
  - Reduce self-criticism, self-isolation, and self-absorption

Singer, T., & Bolz, M. (Eds.). (2013). Compassion: Bridging practice and science. Leipzig: Max Planck Institute for Human Cognitive and Brain Sciences.

Chapter 12

Your Brain on Mindfulness

" The best way to capture moments is to pay attention. This is how we cultivate mindfulness. Mindfulness means being awake. It means knowing what you are doing."
-Jon Kabat-Zinn

We know what we need to know about the wounding. Good work! Now that we have all this excellent knowledge about the problems let's take a further step towards some solutions. Part III has several goals. First, we need some definitions so clear and precise that you'll be able to intelligently discuss the effects on the brain while you're on the treadmill with your recovery buddy before mindfully walking to the hot tub for some soothing self-care. Mainly, you will understand how your brain works when healing practices are applied.

Another job of this section, even if you just skim it, is to give you a felt sense of how seriously awesome and beneficial these principles and practices will be in your life. The practice of making meaning is integral to Compassionate Recovery. To have meaning and purpose may be an everyday thing for many, but for addicts, it has the added benefit of being a lifesaving survival skill. Look for meaning in everything. It matters. It also changes your brain and makes you feel better. Many of us feel ambiguous about everything but our addiction. That changes now.

As you learn to regulate yourself in the twists and turns on the path of recovery, you'll be actively engaged in connecting with and benefit others in whatever community you find yourself in.

This is the last of the brain material. Don't worry; it's brief. The previous chapters on addiction and trauma laid out a basic brain groundwork for our understanding. Fortunately, or unfortunately, the research on these contemplative practices isn't as easy to understand. There isn't a ton of consensus as the field of applied science of mindfulness is relatively new. That said, it's revealed that there are very complex networks of circuits that light up when we use these methods. It would be beyond the scope of this book to go point by point through the research and define too much terminology, but we will add some

Next, you'll read what you need to know about how these brain circuits are affected by practice and how they can be learned. Learning and practicing the use of these circuits leads to healing and well-being. It is because they can be learned that significant effects have been consistently found in the research labs as time goes on. That means you can learn them and apply them to your life.

In Part IV, you'll learn to bring this onto your path of recovery-self-mastery, as we'll focus exclusively on the application of the knowledge that you've worked so hard to attain. You will learn how to practice mindfulness to discern within yourself the differences between different states of empathy, compassion, and self-compassion. As you discover the unbelievable potential of compassion in you, your practice also works at the community level. Let's acquire some more super cool information that we can add to our recovery database.

Mindfulness

Our definition of mindfulness is non-judgmental, present moment awareness of experiences. The bottom line for us is that we can be mindful of our bullshit or mindful of the good shit. It's a personal decision. That said, the discipline of mindfulness originated in Buddhism as a contemplative practice that became the basis for an ethical and ultimately compassionate life. As the foundation of the path to liberate oneself and all beings from suffering, the concentration skills and deep insights gained from mastery of mindfulness led the practitioner beyond the individual to the broader universe of beings who are suffering and need compassion. Because there are over 2500 years of teachings on mindfulness, we can find specific and detailed breakdowns of techniques, insights, and stages of development. For our purposes, we'll keep it simple, smartie.

The application of attention to a specific object of focus, such as your left pinky toe, is to put your mind fully on one thing. We focus our awareness entirely on one point to exclude all else. This is the first step. When we practice such focused attention, we use that focus to widen our awareness which develops a fuller mind, leading to more wisdom. When we're mindful, our mind is full of the object of meditation. Ultimately this focus on one point becomes an open awareness of all matters.

Researchers need specific, operational definitions to distinguish the effect of one variable, the practice of mindfulness, for example, on another variable, the rate of breathing perhaps. The literature on the neuroscience of mindfulness uses the following operational definitions that ensure everyone is measuring the same causes and effects.

In the middle of the last century, scientific inquiry into mindfulness became part of psychotherapy to relieve psychological distress and improve our emotional dimension. These days it is integral to many new approaches. Some of these are MBSR, Mindfulness-Based Stress Reduction, ACT or

Acceptance and Commitment Therapy, and DBT or Dialectical Behavior Therapy, to name a few[82].

These specialized, evidence-based, therapeutic disciplines effectively treat some of our familiar friends: anxiety, depression, PTSD, and addiction, among others. All of this is possible because mindfulness teaches us first to focus, then discern and regulate our emotional states. This comes in handy for those who get overwhelmed or underwhelmed, as it improves a sense of wellness, reduces our emotional hypersensitivity and anxiety, and sharpens our thought process.

Neuroscience of Mindfulness

We learn to notice and discern our tendencies, traits, habits, and patterns through rigorous mindfulness practice. If you've read the chapters in order, this is good stuff for people on the attachment-addiction spectrum. Once we're aware of the more subtle aspects of our humanity, we have an opportunity to make positive changes. In the next section, we'll talk more about integrating mindfulness into recovery on a day to day, moment-by-moment basis.

---

[82] Wheeler, M.S., Arnkoff, D.B. & Glass, C.R. The Neuroscience of Mindfulness: How Mindfulness Alters the Brain and Facilitates Emotion Regulation.

Here, we need to know more about the systems rather than the complex networks of neurons and conflicting theories of the brain that are thought to be involved in mindfulness. To refresh your brain matter on brain matter that we've already covered, e.g., the Prefrontal Cortex and the Amygdala, please refer to Chapter 9. We'll cover only the effects of our contemplative practices rather than repeat material.

You need to know that you can learn mindful practices that train your mind to emotionally self-regulate. That means you are the trainer, and your mind is the trainee. This training, known to monks for thousands of years and now studied in the research labs, improves our most fundamental psychological capacities. All the practices in this book are dose-related. The more mindfulness that you practice, the more mindful you will be. Anyone can do it. That means you.

One of the central circuitries that mindfulness practice improves is attention, or the ability to concentrate on one thing for long periods without distractions. For many of us, our emotional life is very distracting. Financial and relationship problems build up. Attention as a learned skill builds the ability to discern conflicting information. It also helps us monitor how we're doing as we work on problems. What's important about learning the acquired skill of attention is that it influences an increased capacity to regulate our emotional states.

Can you think of three ways this would be helpful in recovery?

With less excitement in our triggered brains, we learn to gain deeper self-awareness over time. We realize this because we train ourselves, our minds. The same reward system that sucks us into the addiction sinkhole can be repurposed or returned to its original intention to help the brain develop and evolve. When we take control, we gain agency of executive function in the frontal lobes. That means clearer thinking and better decisions. The possibilities are endless.

A key takeaway is that mindfulness alone can trigger high ACE people. Therefore, we must have support, actively process what comes up for us, and learn to integrate the results of our deep work into daily life in recovery. That's the entire point of this book.

Let's look at some of the primary brain systems that are enhanced by mindfulness practice[83]. We'll begin with the anterior cingulate cortex.

ACC

At the front of the brain, the anterior cingulate cortex is responsible for many important things for us in our recovery. It's where complex processes

---

[83] Tang YY, Hölzel BK, Posner MI. The neuroscience of mindfulness meditation. Nat Rev Neurosci. 2015 Apr;16(4):213-25

occur, such as impulse control, emotions, decision making, and empathy, which we discuss in detail. You need to know that the ACC is where self-regulation happens, primarily in the areas of the ability to attend to one point of focus and regulation of our ever-troubling emotional content. The ACC enables attention and executive control.

Executive functions control our high-level controls such as memory, inhibition, and flexibility. The brain's executive circuitry, which primarily consists of the prefrontal cortex, allows us to think, plan, solve problems, imagine the future, manage our emotions and impulses, remember our highest values and goals, and make thoughtful decisions.

The executive circuitry allows us to direct our attention where we choose, based on our goals and plans, rather than where it's automatically pulled by internal feelings, thoughts, images, or external sights, sounds, and other stimuli. These are all known as executive functions. This circuitry is connected to other circuitries as it plays a role in emotional experience and behavior, especially in relationships. When we feel safe and have enough support from others and enough skills, we can use our prefrontal cortex to notice, reflect upon, understand, tolerate, and manage painful and unwanted feelings in ourselves and others.

Executive functions also help us resist and overcome unhealthy attachments and impulses, such as those which create incentive salience. Some parts, called self-regulation capacities, play central roles in our capacity to attune to others and relate to them in healthy and fulfilling ways[84]. We need these self-regulatory executive functions to be sharp and healthy to heal from the effects of ACEs and become free of addictions.

We can develop and increase executive functions primarily through our relationships with other people. For example, we first learned how to manage\not manage our fears and cravings from how our parents managed\didn't manage theirs and how they related to our emotions and behaviors. Those meaningful relationships determine the capacities and habits of our executive circuitry.

Unfortunately, traumatic experiences, especially in early childhood and some intoxicating substances, can harm the executive circuitry. Fortunately, because the human brain has an amazing capacity to rewire and heal, such damage is only temporary in most cases. It can be overcome by what is called compensatory brain adaptations. Consider these neuroadaptations that we are in control of. Addiction and trauma caused their own, but now we make new adaptations.

Most importantly, the brain's executive circuitry can be harnessed to bring healing and happiness. We can learn and practice skills for working with our attention, observing, accepting, and transforming

---

[84] This is the main focus of Dan Siegel's interpersonal neurobiology.

our feelings, thoughts, and impulses, and deliberately cultivating healthy and fulfilling habits of thinking, feeling, and behaving.

Amygdala

The amygdala, we know, is central to the limbic system and our emotional processing. In those of us with trauma-related disorders such as we covered earlier, the alarm system is going on, even when there is no external stressor. Guess what happens when we practice the discipline of mindful presence in all our affairs? That's right. The amygdala decreases in activation. It slows down the firing of stress hormones. Fight or flight calms down. Freeze becomes a free flow.

What other super brain powers does mindfulness teach us? This is a cool one. It decreases our anxiety about ourselves and reduces our negative beliefs about ourselves. A good practice would be to discuss this with someone in recovery. Please spread the word that we can reduce our negative, fear-based emotional anxiety by affecting our brains with intentional, consistent practice. When emotional images flash before us, we're as calm as a mountain lake.

PFC

Our central processing unit, the prefrontal cortex, regulates attention and emotion. Aside from the clarity of renewed attention, the PFC also reacts better to control emotions in mindful meditators. These parts light up more and more on the imaging as practice develops. It connects with the amygdala and facilitates a reduction in feelings of anxiety.

PCC

The posterior cingulate cortex is connected to the thalamus and is an important part of the midbrain processing of sensory data, which runs through our limbic system. It's part of the upper limbic lobe and is where the formation of emotions and processing, learning, and memory occurs.

It's also part of the seat of self-awareness. During meditation, the PCC slows down. That means our emotional state loosens as our perception increases and awareness deepens. These are good reasons to take the life practice seriously.

Insula

The insula is also associated with emotional processing, but its role in self-awareness is more important. The fascinating thing about it is that when we practice mindfulness consistently over time, it thickens our brain, sharpens our internal and external focus, and gives us a chance to regulate our emotions. The insula is also the place where awareness becomes aware of itself. In the history of homo sapiens, this is the defining factor and the cause of the cognitive revolution that led us where we are today. If we have experiences of non-duality or pure, raw experience like a basket of joy and grounded fascination that holds all the suffering of humanity in its palms, this is the place in the brain where that happens.

It's about present moment awareness and our interactions on physical, mental, emotional, and spiritual dimensions, the meanings we ascribe, decisions we make, and actions we take. When we meditate, the insula lights up, paving the road for insight into the more profound Wisdom of Compassion.

Let me caution you. If you're a traumatized individual like me, you may have an experience similar to mine and that of most people I've met in recovery. We spend our lives running from the ongoing stress NTs juicing up our poor emotional brain. We do this with our attachments and addictions. When we sit still, the vibes may be too intense. In decades of mindful practice, I had quite a few Complex PTSD experiences without much psychological or emotional support from the meditation community. It was difficult, as I always felt like a raw nerve, and everyone expected me to be calm after meditation. My experience was quite the opposite!

Here's some good news. When meditators follow their mindfulness training with compassion training, they don't trip. Things are calm. Connections are open. This is a point that I don't think can be overemphasized. When we live in the capacity of avoiding pain, then open ourselves up to the wound, we need medicine ready. That medicine is your empathy, self-compassion, and compassion for others. We'll get there in the next section. I just want those who feel triggered when they sit still to know that you're not alone. It's OK. You can do it.

Another fascinating aspect of our ability to directly affect our insula through strategic target practice is changing the reference point of who we think we are. This self-referencing is opened up, freed, and expanded by being *compassionately* aware of itself. You need to know that your narrative, the story you have about yourself, told by caregivers and yourself, well, you're the boss of changing that story. Write a new sober script, as I mentioned earlier. The important key takeaway here is that you can be the author of your own story. That factor is key to the primary therapeutic interventions for trauma in that we learn to have the confidence to write our own stories. As I've said, you're the boss. Talk about this in a meeting or with your circle of safety. Make a social media post asking what people think about it. Expand your circle of like-minded folks. Not everyone will be on the same page, but when you find the gold nuggets of common ground with a few people, it will be worth all the not-as-good nuggets that we may come across.

Striatum

This part of the brain that is heavily influenced by mindful practice is part of a complex group of brain structures with many names that we don't need to know for our purposes. It enables us to make smooth, coordinated moves towards something of interest. The striatum is connected to a nucleus of cells known to be involved in our reward system. Here's what's critical. The striatum is active between the urge to get some of our addiction and the compulsion to go after it. It's another area involved in incentive salience or the anticipation of anything that we find pleasurable.

This circuit calms down in meditators.

Mindfulness activates parts of the striatum that facilitate emotional regulation and our friend attention. When our mind is chill, the regulation happens automatically in what has been called in the research setting a resting state. We, addicts, need a resting state and a deeper than the average person relaxation and letting go of attachment. That means mindfulness is good practice for us.

Another reason is that the striatum is associated with the basal ganglia and the mesolimbic dopamine reward system. When we're in our addiction, the NTs involved with the addictive process of incentive salience go on blast until we're hooked like a monkey in a banana tree. We see something; the cerebral cortex decides it's interesting and passes a signal over to the basal ganglia; part of the energy goes out to the striatum to create contiguous moves towards the thing we're after.

When we practice mindfulness and apply it in times of urgency, all that cools down. Nice.

Bottoms Up!

The way we process information is conceptualized as top-down or bottom-up. In top-down, prefrontal, cognitive data passes down into the midbrain, extended amygdala, and the whole limbic system.

In bottom-up processing, the raw sensory data is processed deep in the older parts of the brain, then to the intellectual centers for meaning-making. We can make new, positive, compassionate meaning if we know how to use this process.

Bottom-up healing practices focus on embodying the physical experience rather than a cognitive emphasis, such as Peter Levine's Somatic Experiencing therapy for PTSD. We'll continue with our theme that promotes practices like yoga, t'ai chi, and martial arts because most clinicians recognize these as key to healing trauma and addiction.

The top-down clinical approach is to reframe your thoughts about the experience that you're having. You tell yourself positive things and talk yourself out of your bad feelings. But with bottom-up, you acknowledge and allow yourself to embrace the experience in the body. This releases traumatic emotional energy, but it is a process that takes time and a multi-faceted approach. The principles and practices of Compassionate Recovery support the approach from the top, bottom, and sideways. Whatever promotes our healing is on the menu.

Some researchers feel that mindfulness practice is bottom-up, while others say it's top-down. In a survey of mindfulness literature, researchers found that even short-term mindfulness practice reduced reactivity to complex emotional stimuli, increased mental stability, and improved over time with practice. A more top-down is used in the beginning stages because we use language to learn the technique. We need the PFC to understand instructions and monitor progress.

Over time, the practice of mindfulness affects deeper regions of the brain that are beyond words. As you know, the feeling of no separation or universal connectedness is in the insula. This is what is meant by a felt sense. Within us, these are feeling spaces rather than mental. The practices of somatic awareness combined with mindfulness increase the brain's ability to be more aware. We train our minds to handle better and better[85].

These processes of top-down and bottom-up are intertwined and interact in complex ways. They're not always separate things. Understanding this as a

---

85 -Clin Psychol Rev. 2013 Feb;33(1):82-96. doi: 10.1016/j.cpr.2012.10.006. Mindfulness: top-down or bottom-up emotion regulation strategy? Chiesa, Serretti, Jakobsen

framework for healing is sufficient. We should always work with the words and the feelings while understanding these distinct yet related processes.

Integration Practice: Flip the Mindfulness Switch

Once you flip the right switches, our neurotransmitters will deliver the results that we need instead of those that are unhealthy. We're informed about what goes on within us; now, we can do something that immediately begins to create benefit. Flip the switch of mindful compassion on and keep it on with consistent practice.

Sit in your meditation position. Decide what you're going to be mindful of. In this case, we'll choose the rising and falling of the belly as you breathe. Decide that you're going to focus on this alone. Make that commitment for 10 minutes. Your mind will drift off the belly on to something else, like what you want to put in your belly. We notice our distraction and gently bring our attention, using all the brain parts that we just learned about, to the object of meditation. We get lost, then catch ourselves and return. In Buddhism, this is called vigilance. It's about keeping a watchful eye on your mind, trillion quintillion times, or however long it takes to untie the knots that snare us. Be mindful. Be vigilant. Repeat until there is no one to be aware of and nothing to be cognizant of, no matter how long that takes.

Notes

Chapter 13
Your Brain on Empathy

> *"The crucial distinction between the term empathy and those like sympathy, empathic concern, and compassion is that empathy denotes that the observer's emotions reflect affective sharing or 'feeling with' the other person while compassion, sympathy, empathic concern denote that the observer's emotions are inherently other oriented or 'feeling for' the other person".*[86]
> -Tania Singer, PhD

A baby looks up at its mother and automatically learns to mimic the emotional expressions on her face, vocal sounds, and other movements. This is called *mimicry* in the research and is the first function on a spectrum of empathy. It allows us to understand and share each other's emotional humanity automatically. There is a direct relationship between mimicry and a

---

[86] Singer T, Lamm C. The social neuroscience of empathy. Ann N Y Acad Sci. 2009 Mar;1156:81-96

baseline of empathy. It's the first layer of brain function in the process of empathic concern.

It's the crack of dawn, and one of the chickens starts squawking. Before long, the whole coop is squawking along with the same tone and rhythm. They feel the distress of the other bird, but they don't have any way to make a cognitive determination of the reason for the distress and therefore aren't able to unlink from the original distress. This is called *emotional contagion* in the neuroscience of emotion literature. It's not yet empathy, but it's a required step along the spectrum.

Empathy, from the Greek *en pathos* or in passion, is what we experience when we experience someone else's emotional experience. First, we recognize their distress. Then we feel the same despair until we check the other person and realize, "OK, that's how they're feeling; I'm just resonating with their emotional reality in this moment." If we don't make that distinction, it's easy to get into an allostatic overload spiral of toxic, emotionally negative kaka.

Why do we need to learn about and practice empathy in recovery? Imagine a world without empathy. What if everyone were their own autocrat, and nobody felt anything when others suffered? While we don't necessarily consider empathy and how it works in our brains, it's impossible to find common humanity without it. We remain isolated in our shrinking world without common humanity—when we're in our addiction. We're no longer isolated, alienated, and resentful when we're in our recovery. Instead, we feel the warmth inside ourselves and with others. We're curious and empathetic to others which becomes the basis for enduring friendship and lifetime support in recovery. Let's not underestimate the foundation of our well-being.

This basis of empathic brain processes goes back to about a hundred million years. The palaeomammalian brain is more or less the same as the limbic system in its function, particularly all the oxytocin goodness that happens when we connect on a genuine level with another warm-blooded being.

The first two levels of mimicry and emotional contagion themselves can't account for the total experience of empathy. In the last section on mindfulness, we talked about attention as a learned skill in meditation. Through the insula, a self-reference or self-awareness exists, even to the point of awareness being aware of itself or you watching you be your best you[87].

This attention from our mindfulness practice can be applied to a critical aspect of empathy which is discrete from mimicry and emotion contagion, which is discernment. We need to learn how not to own other people's feelings. Do you think that should be a key takeaway? Talk about it with

---

[87] Baby steps.

someone. How often do you take on the emotional experience of people whose experience you'd rather not have? Journal about this.

We can and must learn to discern or distinguish between the distress in another and ourselves as two separate things. Otherwise, we can spiral. Any addict knows the emotional spiral, and those with ACEs have been in it deeply. Therefore, this idea of being able to discern our emotional responsibility from someone else is a key factor in developing ourselves into a happy person in Compassionate Recovery. We do it with new narratives, focused meditations, and directed practices on our own and in community.

When we practice empathy, especially mindfulness, our self-awareness circuits get brighter and stronger. It becomes easier to tell who's feeling what in a particular situation which used to be baffling. If we did have this ability, our experience might turn into personal distress and require a more self-centered reaction than one would consider empathetic. It's also possible that empathic responses can trigger us. This may be a reason to withdraw, both internally and socially—time to change that.

Sympathy is distinct from empathy but is built on it. It doesn't involve feelings of sadness but is an emotionally concerning connection. As we may have discovered by now, compassion is the feeling of suffering *with* another, combined with the need to take action to alleviate their suffering. This formula leads to altruism, or benevolent, selfless action. Social neuroscientists call it pro-social behavior. But it's just kindness, isn't it?

Empathy leads to compassion which leads to compassionate action. These actions lead to unbelievable benefits for the person giving and those receiving. These skills are broken up into thinking and feeling aspects in many trainings available to anyone interested. We can learn to put ourselves in someone else's shoes with empathy, then learn to experience deeper connectivity and mental health through compassion that leads us to volunteering, donating, and taking care of others. Please be forewarned, however. With all that we know about how our brains learn to get attached to things, we can get hooked on this compassion business. Research shows that the more empathy we practice, the more compassionate we become, and the more compassionate we become, the more good things we do.

It's the un-vicious cycle.

Neuroscience of Empathy

According to some researchers, mirror neurons play a significant role in empathic responses. They are the most hyped brain cell, as they're thought to be pivotal to our understanding of social cognition, or how we analyze social interactions constantly for survival and learning. We mimic, connect, gain trust, understand emotion, build trust in others, and learn to be in the world as part of the social fabric of family and community. As children, we learn how to be in the world from our caregivers. But context matters. We're all growed up now and are taking responsibility for our own healing. We can make new brain cells, patterns, and lovely experiences with ourselves and other beings is learnable and enhanceable because it's dose-related.

Remember, there are people in the world who have cognitive empathy but are missing the circuits for emotional empathy. They can be narcissists who use empathic people for their amusement and feel nothing about it. But they can trick us, take advantage, or even imprison and torture us because they know what to say to make us feel understood. If we're dealing with a malignant narcissist, they only know what they need to use us.

They intellectually understand what empathy is and how you're supposed to look and act if you have empathy because mirror neurons—duh. Some of us may have grown up in situations of abuse where the caregiver was devoid of emotional empathy. We need to learn it and be an expression of empathic joy in the world, despite being bird food for emotional vultures. We still get to exist to our fullest capacities.

Cognitive Empathy

This aspect of our empathic connection to living beings is the part that knows intellectually that others have an experience, be it joy or pain. On the mental dimension, we take on someone's energy by seeing the world through their eyes, at least at that moment. This helps us create a context or framework for understanding that person. If we've never put much effort into this, it will take time to develop. But if we think about our connection with others with these things in mind, we empower ourselves with incredible meaning and purpose. If we only have the cognitive aspect, there is no vicarious experience of the other person's feelings; it's just an idea. It's a notion that's necessary but not sufficient for the whole empathy experience.

Neuroscience of Cognitive Empathy

There are several brain systems reflected in the research. Most are prefrontal cortex-related areas that are involved in this function. We need to know about the temporoparietal unction or TPJ. This circuit allows us to differentiate the emotional experience as belonging to the other person. We know we can feel it, but we don't have to own it. The pain is real, but it's not ours.

Emotional Empathy

Yo, I feel you. Loosely translated, this means my mirror neurons are kicking in. I feel like I understand how you feel, like mentally and so forth, and I'm sure that you and I are sharing an isomorphic or very similar experience! This is called affective empathy, experience sharing, and is through to be defined by the fact that a) we're experiencing the same feelings, b) the reason we're experiencing those feelings is that we were triggered by the other person's experience and c) we can feel this in our body. In recovery, we call it a gut-level response.

Neuroscience of Affective Empathy

When subjects view someone else experiencing suffering, the brain's parts that light up are the anterior midcingulate cortex or aMCC and the aI or anterior insula. You'll recall the insula's function earlier in mindfulness. Here, we have a particular kind of mindfulness called salience or clarity. If we experience personal distress resulting from an empathic overload triggered by someone else, these areas bring it all into very sharp focus. We may have a negative experience of empathy and prefer to live behind our walls of aloneness. We're done with that now, however. With our mindfulness and other practices, we will learn to accurately discern our emotions in ourselves and know what is ours. Then we can reserve deeper empathic connections with others that are people that we trust and deserve our confidence in them to be empathetic to us.

Empathy and Emotional Regulation

Suppose our empathy is going to lead to compassionate and beneficial actions toward our inner selves and our communities. In that case, we need to have the skill of emotional regulation, which we've discussed throughout the book thus far. It's key to our development on the path of recovery to self-mastery, on whatever levels of mastery we aspire to; mental, physical, emotional, or spiritual. If we're emotionally out of control, our relationships crumble with ourselves and each other. We're talking here about learning to regulate instead of being regulated by our traumas and addictions.

The fact is that people who can regulate their feelings are more likely to engage in the critical second half of compassion, namely the compulsion to act to relieve suffering.

We did this with our addiction to relieve suffering when we jumped on the needle or the spoon and took our trip to the moon. But we can repurpose this circuitry and intentionally train ourselves to jump just as fast and twice as high to benefit others. That's a feeling you can't get in powder form. And it's one that the literature shows us that we can make a new mind map whenever we want to. People who use techniques like thinking about situations differently or cognitive restructuring tend to be more proactive in the field of compassionate action. Be one of these.

However, we do need to use our empathy boundaries to protect ourselves from toxic energy. That means that our regulation skills are helpful for turning on empathy and turning it off when needed. That's the definition of emotional regulation. We're in control, not our wild, trauma-based neurology.

We're discussing all of these separately, but on a moment-by-moment basis within our vast neural universe, the processes of mindfulness, empathy, self-compassion, and compassion are inseparable. That's good news because the practices all support each other, which means we are supported in our recovery, our Compassionate Recovery.

Integration Practice: Trip the Empathy Trigger

Find a place to rest your mind. Use mindfulness to get there, though there is not a place one can arrive at. Learn to discern one feeling in your body that you know is yours. This may take coming back several or many times. It might take years. But the goal is to discern your feelings from other people's. The first step is a consistent, daily mindfulness practice. There are so many options and apps and zooms, and you name it. Get on that for yourself. Make it work. Develop the skill to know how you feel. Then in your meditation, ask, "Do I know how I feel? How do I feel?"

As you proceed on this path, ask yourself this question. Ask it in your meditation. Inquire with every being that you encounter throughout your journey. The object of your study is the following question, "Do I *know* how they feel? Do I *feel* how they feel?"

Write about this process. Get a separate Empathy Journal. Work on this with someone else or a small group in recovery. Make it fun. Go on walks together in nature. Bring pets and kids. Be a community empath in recovery.

Notes

Chapter 14
Your Brain on Self-compassion

"Instead of mercilessly judging and criticizing yourself for various inadequacies or shortcomings, self-compassion means you are kind and understanding when confronted with personal failings."
-Kristen Neff, PhD

Christians, Buddhists, and many other traditions have taught that we should have compassion for others for thousands of years. The Tibetan Buddhists have a litany of step-by-step practices to develop compassion for others. These practices, such as mindfulness, loving-kindness, compassion, empathic joy, equanimity, and tonglen or exchanging self for others, are now mainstream in clinical research and practice for trauma and addiction. You'll be hard-pressed to find a respectable treatment provider who hasn't been trained in some variation of these practices.

Over the past few decades, I've received sets of complex instructions on the subject of compassion from different masters, including the Dalai Lama. Much of my understanding was merely a form of cognitive empathy rather than genuine compassion. But it takes what it takes to learn what we need to learn if we're lucky enough to learn it at all, and I'm a slow learner. To practice compassion for others, I would have to get over the hurdle of a lifetime of self-criticism. As a beneficiary and supporter of psychotherapy, it became obvious that I'd need an integrated solution to apply compassion to myself. That led me to Mindful Self-compassion, or MSC, a 10-week course created by Chris Germer, Ph.D., and Dr. Kristen Neff.

The concept of practicing self-compassion is relatively new in the psychological literature. Dr. Neff is the psychologist who pioneered the concept of self-compassion in modern psychology based on her interest in Buddhism and meditation. In 2003 she published the first Self-compassion scale[88] ever used in the field. The first time I took the test, my score was 1.88, which is very low on the Self-compassion scale. But the good news is that Self-compassion isn't a static measure. We can change it with practice. It's dose-dependent or dose-related, as

---

88 Neff, K. D. (2003). Development and validation of a scale to measure self-compassion. *Self and Identity, 2*, 223-250. I recommend that you take your Self-compassion test now and return to it regularly as a form of self-examination. Remember, the results change and are dose related. https://self-compassion.org/test-how-self-compassionate-you-are/

are the other practices. Do more of it, get better at it. Get addicted to feeling connected with yourself and your community. What does practice help you get better at?

You will learn to be comfortable in your own skin. The practice of Self-compassion is at the core of my recovery. I've learned to be at ease within myself in ways that I never imagined. But it wasn't easy to learn this practice. It is not my default state. It takes consistent effort to apply the principles and practices. But they are 100% worth it and always pay off.

After taking MSC and the Cultivating Compassion course from Stanford University's Compassion Institute, I was surprised at how much these secular, evidence-based trainings added to my years of experience with meditation. It took two rounds of MSC to break my wall of self-loathing, but I eventually learned how to practice self-compassion, little by little, until I could feel it and make it part of my recovery.

These tools work without needing to be Buddhist. But if you practice them, you couldn't be more Buddhist. And you don't even need a hat.

Self-compassion for me needed to be cracked open and integrated into my life so that compassion for others could flourish. It may work differently for you. Some people are compassionate by nature; the rest of us must work at it. The benefits of this opening can't be overstated. It's absolutely life-changing once it starts to flow.

We learn to notice and discern when we're being self-critical and how to replace it with loving kindness toward ourselves. Self-care and self-soothing become part of our natural response to our stress. This is where we learn about humanity that we all share. To the addict, this profound experience is key to ending the isolation that keeps us apart rather than a part of.

Once we begin to see that we're part of the human experience, which is flawed, but we're not, our reactions are more understandable. We start to see that we make sense, even if we want to change some things. We're not as confused about who we are, so we free up that part of us that creates a new, self-empowered narrative. We don't have to identify with our traumas and addictions. There's a freedom to choose how we want to see ourselves.

Practices in Compassionate Recovery are geared toward freedom that includes the ability to stay in our window of tolerance and out of the funnel. That means we need to learn how to tolerate painful emotions without escaping. Self-compassion is the inroad for this ability. It must be used with mindfulness, don't forget that.

As we learned earlier, toxic stress is at the core of our suffering. Self-compassion teaches us to calm down the fight or flight circuits, taming the output of adrenaline, cortisol, and other stress hormones. It opens us up to the same nurturing oxytocin that our mothers would give us. Natural pain relief flows when the knots of self-confusion caused by trauma and addiction loosen. Mindfulness provides us with the chance to catch it while it's happening and make new circuits our default.

Self-compassion has been shown in the lab to reduce depression and anxiety and shame, and suicidal tendencies. Conversely, our self-compassionate mind state spills over into other cool mind states like happiness and self-confidence. Are you sold on self-compassion yet?

It will lead you to a feeling of well-being and connectedness. But remember, self-compassion isn't the same as self-esteem, which is mainly about our worth and standing and a leaning toward narcissistic tendencies. Self-compassion is more like holding a newborn baby swaddled in a blanky than building yourself up for the corporate hurdles.

You will feel better and won't get sick as often. This is also true of yoga and other amazing physical wellness activities that you are totally going to get into, right? People who have higher self-compassion heal more quickly from PTSD, so it follows that we can apply self-compassion to heal our trauma.

Put your hand on your heart and say, "It's OK." Feel the warmth. Smile. It's OK, really.

When we integrate mindfulness and self-compassion into our recovery, we will be more confident and less terrified of failure. In case you were wondering, the literature also reveals that self-compassion is linked to reduced eating disorders, better relationships, and, wait for it...reduction in addictive drives.

Neuroscience of Self-compassion[89]

There isn't a vast amount of research yet in the area of self-compassion, as we find in addiction and trauma, but the field is growing. We know that the practice thickens our gray matter, called GMV for gray matter volume. You'll remember that mindfulness also causes an increase in the volume of the insula.

The ACC, directly influencing emotional regulation, also grows with self-compassion. Think about this in comparison to how addiction works. The more addicted we get, the more addicted we get. The secret of this whole book is learning to retool your existing brain circuits to build a loving and extraordinary life. The practice of self-compassion alone does the same thing, except that the more self-compassion we practice, the more self-

---

[89] Guan, F., Liu, G., Pedersen, W. S., Chen, O., Zhao, S., Sui, J., & Peng, K. (2021). Neurostructural correlates of dispositional self-compassion. Neuropsychologia, 160, 107978.

compassionate we become. We beef up our ACC and load up on oxytocin while learning to chill instead of panicking at every feeling.

A region in the prefrontal lobes called the dorsolateral prefrontal cortex, or DLPFC, plays a role in executive function, including short-term memory and other attention-oriented tasks, which, as we know, are also enhanced by mindfulness practice. We need to understand that an integrated mindful, self-compassionate life path clears our mind to make nicer decisions, based on altruistic intentions that make better connections, meaning, and purpose. This is where recovery lives, not in a church basement talking about how different we are from everyone else. Look for the similarities or common humanity.

We begin to see ourselves in intellectually and emotionally clear ways instead of the distorted lens of addiction or the shame of child abuse. We can empathize with ourselves, which means that our empathy circuits are interconnected with our self-esteem circuits.

Let's light 'em up!

Integration Practice: Turn Up the Volume of Self-compassion

Along with your regular, consistent mindfulness practice, learn to listen in silence. Allow your whole being to absorb the energy of sound vibrations as if every pore were a pair of ears. Be as still as a clear pond at the top of a mountain on a windless day. Listen to the softest and the furthest sounds without analysis, categorization, or a decision about good or bad, pleasant or unpleasant. Get into the Zen of Sound. Being just this moment, as it is.

Now that you're developing the skill of getting into this mind space use it to listen to your innermost voices. Think about your ACEs, your family, school, and community experiences. Allow yourself to feel what addiction has been like for you from a calm, self-regulated state.

Put your hand on your heart and say, "It's OK," because it is, and you are. Do this practice every morning when you put your feet on the floor. Take two or three minutes to listen to your self-compassion heartbeat. The way to turn up the volume and hear it more clearly is to get out of the way. Your care for you is in there. It's what got you here.

Extra credit: read Part II of this book with a friend or group of friends in recovery. Discuss your own experiences. Practice supporting each other in learning self-compassion. Remember, no caretaking! We take care of each other by taking care of ourselves.

Notes

Chapter 15
Your Brain on Compassion

"The word compassion derives from the Latin expression compati, meaning literally to suffer with. Considered among all of the world's major religious traditions as one of the most cherished of virtues, compassion is widely accepted as a sensitivity to the suffering of another and a desire to alleviate that suffering."
-Larry Stevens, C. Chad Woodruff [90]

From the perspective of social psychology, compassion is its own separate and distinct state. But it's not one thing; it's rather complex and involves more than one system. We feel things when we see someone suffering or in need, but compassion isn't just an emotion. It evokes emotions such as sadness, love, or a mix. Nor is compassion the same as sympathy because

---

[90] Editor(s): Larry Stevens, C. Chad Woodruff, The Neuroscience of Empathy, Compassion, and Self-Compassion, Academic Press, 2018 and Goetz, J. L., Keltner, D., & Simon-Thomas, E. (2010). Compassion: An evolutionary analysis and empirical review. Psychological Bulletin, 136(3), 351–374

sympathy and its cousin pity aren't motivated by empathetic connection and the motivation to do something about it. Compassion isn't love but is related to love and is part of love. Compassionate love has been defined in the literature as

"...*an attitude toward others, either close others or strangers or all of humanity; containing feelings, cognitions, and behaviors that are focused on caring, concern, tenderness, and an orientation toward supporting, helping, and understanding the others, particularly when the others are perceived to be suffering or in need.*[91]"

Compassion has been defined in numerous ways across different fields in which we can educate ourselves. But to be honest, it's not something that a group of words on paper will make us understand. No matter how many brilliant people have written on the topic, it's like describing a love song. Just sing the damn thing so we can feel something! So, we learn to listen to our hearts in mindful silence as we understand on the mental, emotional, physical, and spiritual levels what the Light of Compassion is as a way of being rather than a mere idea about being. The song of compassion must be sung for its music that must be felt.

It took us a while to get here. I appreciate your patience and dedication to healing for reading all the

---

[91] *Sprecher & Fehr (2005), cited in Goetz (2010)*

preceding chapters. If you skip around, that's fine too, because all roads lead to compassion. But to get on the road, we need a decent vehicle to take us out of the suffering of holding ourselves up against the pressures of the world into a life of meaning, purpose, connection, and joyful service.

This is the last chapter in the story of your brain on trauma, addiction, and contemplative healing practices. We'll put the knowledge to work in the next section as we craft our path. To finish this part of the book, we need to know where compassion is experienced in us and how it affects our healing in recovery. Remember that we can train in and improve on our compassion skill set. It works if you work it.

Neuroscience of Compassion

In empathy, we use emotional recognition, comprehension, and resonance with the other person or people. Still, compassion adds the ability to tolerate our gut reaction and the necessary component of compassion, the motivation to get our feet moving urgently to help relieve suffering[92].

If empathy emerges on a spectrum, compassion is the pot of gold at the end of the neurological rainbow. In empathy, we must differentiate between our feelings and another's, but we also need to

---

92 Mindfulness (N Y). 2018 June ; 9(3): 708–724. doi:10.1007/s12671-017-0841-8.

regulate emotionally so that we can transition into compassion, which in and of itself is a self-regulatory function. The more you regulate, the more you regulate. Compassion helps us regulate. Do more practice, be more regular[93].

Compassion differs from empathy in the neural circuitries that are activated[94]. We don't need to go all the way into the other's feeling state for compassion to arise. A little empathy is all that's required to get us into action.

Like the sensitivity we talked about around mindfulness practice, our ACE-related circuits may get triggered when we're empathetic, as we discussed. But the critical point is that the ability to handle that discomfort from the mindfulness is required to get into empathy, which can bring up another level of toxicity that needs to be purged. We must not resist the healing process, but we don't have to do it alone.

The sensitivity exists again in an empathetic response. To know that the other person is in distress and that the empathic distress that we feel is not ours lets us know that someone is suffering or in need and prompts us to act. We need regulation in our emotional brain centers during this process, though it happens instantly. Systematic, consistent training in compassion teaches us to regulate, as it

---

[93] Not in a Metamucil kind of way, sorry.

[94] Tania Singer & Matthias Bolz. "Compassion - Bridging Practice and Science."

shows up on fMRI scans that three main areas of the brain are positively enhanced.

When subjects are trained in a combined practice of cognitive and emotional empathy and compassion skills, compassion becomes the tool that heals on a neuro level. These skills allow us to take care of our emotional reactions to take compassionate action to help someone. Three areas of the brain sometimes referred to as a compassion network, show enhancement in the lab: the ventral striatum or VS, the subgenual or lower anterior cingulate cortex, the sgACC, and the medial orbitofrontal cortex, mOFC. The striatum, as we know, is involved in the reward and pleasure circuitries. The ACC is where we regulate emotions, and the frontal cortex is where intellectual and emotional thinking happens. These are all linked to the limbic system, primarily the amygdala.

The data also shows that activation in these areas is causally related to charitable deeds. Meditate, be a better human. Feel better. Help others. Compassionate Recovery is about training our brain to do all of this. These are our tasks in this model of recovery.

A meta-analysis [95] of the neuro data on compassion reveals the following nine brain

---

95 Editor(s): Larry Stevens, C. Chad Woodruff, The Neuroscience of Empathy, Compassion, and Self-Compassion, Academic Press

regions, most of which we've covered. The emphasis of each is specified in some exciting ways, all of which are upgrades due to compassion training. As we mentioned, the amygdala, or the center of fear, is calmed and regulated—the AI, where we feel disgust and internal sensations, is relaxed. The OFC, usually where anger and internal and external sensations are processed, is eased. The ACC, connected to the compassion network mentioned above, is energized as sadness is replaced with the joy of easing suffering in others.

The dmPFC or dorsomedial prefrontal cortex and the TPF or temporal-parietal junction mentioned previously are involved in the representation of self to self. In the posterior cingulate cortex, PCC lies the ability to discern the experience of self from others and the clarity to think through the emotional experience and make sense of it, rather than being distressed and overwhelmed in a blown-out window of tolerance that might knock us into the funnel. The vlPFC or ventrolateral prefrontal cortex, where we form language to describe the abstract nuance of emotion, is improved. The dlPFC, dorsolateral prefrontal cortex, part of executive function and memory, is upgraded with compassion practice. It is particularly enhanced by cognitive regulation or thinking through the emotional experience of yourself and another. The periaqueductal gray, an emotional arousal adaptation site, thickens as our ability to regulate our emotions improves. Finally, the visual cortex, where we process sight, gets sharper in processing emotional stimuli in ourselves and the faces of others, as in the empathy studies where they tested recognition of emotional states based on facial expressions. This insight allows us to connect with other people and understand how they feel.

The compassion experience involves both top-down and bottom-up processing. We feel through the limbic, emotional brain and think through the prefrontal lobes as we encounter another's suffering, identify our feelings and how they are different, possibly experience varying degrees of empathy, and discern a course of action to help the other person out. It's a whole-brain experience.

Compassion has the potential to heal the whole brain.

Psychopaths: The Opposite of Compassion

Psychopaths. Malignant Narcissists. We all know one. Some of us marry them or grow up with one. Maybe we coincidentally work for one. Do you feel like these types always find you? That may be because they use cognitive without emotional empathy to seek out vulnerable types. According to Scientific American,

"Superficially charming, psychopaths tend to make a good first impression on others and often strike observers as remarkably normal. Yet they are self-centered, dishonest, and undependable, and at times they engage in irresponsible behavior for no apparent reason other than the sheer fun of it. Largely devoid of guilt, empathy, and love, they have casual and callous interpersonal and romantic relationships. Psychopaths routinely offer excuses for their reckless and often outrageous actions, blaming others instead. They rarely learn from their mistakes or benefit from negative feedback, and they have difficulty inhibiting their impulses."

Psychopaths make up about 25% of prison inmates in the US and comprise about 1 in 4 CEOs of US corporations. The psychopaths studied in prisons showed low or no activation in the brain's empathy circuits when subjected to images of others suffering. There are two terms used in the literature. One is imagine-self, where the subject imagines that the pain in the images that are shown is happening to them. Even psychopaths' brains light up in the right places when they do the *imagine-self* exercise— because they're narcissists! Then there's the *imagine-other* version, where they were asked to imagine that the event was happening to another person. Psychopaths don't do well at this one.

In an fMRI study[96], subjects with psychopathy had their pain circuits light up when they took the imagine-self perspective. But when they took the imagine-self point of view, the empathy circuits were as dark as Christmas lights in July.

In addition to dead or offline empathy circuits, the psychopath's pleasure centers light up with images of imagine-other. Yes, that is as scary as it sounds. Psychopaths enjoy the suffering of others.

When it comes to compassion, a psychopath is the opposite of an empath. While they feel no personal distress or affective empathy as they encounter suffering, the empath feels everything. If you're an empath, look out. Some feed on us.

Some scientists claim that psychopathy is treatable and that not all psychopaths are violent. We'll leave that discussion to the professionals. For our purposes in recovery, we can understand that our symptoms are always treatable. Suffering is the symptom. Compassion is healing.

Most psychopaths are male, but it's unclear why that's disproportionate to female psychopaths. According to some clinicians, a true psychopath doesn't have the standard empathy circuits, or at least if they do, they don't function normally. Some of us won't like to hear this, but in addiction, we

---

[96] "An fMRI study of affective perspective taking in individuals with psychopathy: imagining another in pain does not evoke empathy." Decety Jean, Chen Chenyi, Harenski Carla, Kiehl Kent, Frontiers in Human Neuroscience, VOL 7, 2013

might sometimes become something like a temporary psychopath.

I'll use the term *temporary psychopathy* to reflect that, given a particular moment in our addiction, even in recovery, these circuits are still there and can fire up when we fall into some of these mechanisms. This is more likely if we have high ACEs and mental illness. Just because we've acted like a psychopath doesn't mean we are one. But we need to be gut-level honest with ourselves. How often has addiction kept us from honoring the common humanity of others, particularly those we claim to love?

Psychopathy is the official disorder of psychopaths and sociopaths. When we're into addiction, we don't have empathy. As we learned earlier, the chemicals take over our brains, and we at least temporarily stop caring about the harm we cause others. Later, when feelings of empathy do arise, the shame, guilt, and self-loathing are unbearable.

This triggers us into addictive behaviors.

Compassion Fatigue

In the helping professions, and among people like first responders and those of us who are codependent, the phenomenon known as compassion fatigue can take its toll. According to Dr. Charles Figley of the Tulane Traumatology Institute, compassion fatigue is *"a state experienced by those helping people or animals in distress; it is an extreme state of tension and preoccupation with the suffering of those being helped to the degree that it can create a secondary traumatic stress for the helper."*

Note that this is an extreme state of preoccupation. Consider that he's talking about the average person, not hypersensitive trauma survivors. For addicts, the state of focus is our default mode! It's easy for us to get obsessed with almost anything. Note that for myself and most of the addicts I've known, compassion is *not* our default mode. It's a good thing there is professional and spiritual training available.

Compassion fatigue is often confused with empathy fatigue[97]. Empathy fatigue is a state of mental, emotional, physical, and spiritual exhaustion that happens when front-line workers are confronted with non-stop stories of trauma, grief, and loss.

We can all run the risk of empathy and compassion fatigue when we care about and try to help other beings. While we strive to develop empathy and compassion, remember that we all respond differently. Some of us will need to learn how to tone it down rather than ramp it up. Those

---

[97] Empathy Fatigue: Healing the Mind, Body, and Spirit of Professional Counselors, Mark A. Stebnicki (2000, 2001)

who don't feel much compassion or empathy will approach practice differently than those who can't *not* feel it on an overwhelming level.

It's essential to make these distinctions related to our experiences with our addictions. We need to know how we're feeling first, then how to manage distress and being overwhelmed in order to regulate our emotions, build better relationships with ourselves and be of benefit to our community.

It's important to recognize these dysregulations as possible triggers or funnel factors that could send us down a spiral into relapse rather than up the spiral into self-mastery. Dr. Judith Orloff explains how we become empaths,

"Many factors can contribute. Some babies enter the world with more sensitivity than others—an inborn temperament. You can see it when they come out of the womb. They're more responsive to light, smells, touch, movement, temperature, and sound. Also, from what I've observed with my patients and workshop participants, some sensitivity may be genetically transmitted. Highly sensitive children can come from mothers and fathers with the same traits. In addition, parenting plays a role. Childhood neglect or abuse can also affect the sensitivity levels of adults. Many empaths I've treated have experienced early trauma, such as emotional or physical abuse, or were raised by alcoholic, depressed, or narcissistic parents. This could wear down the usual healthy defenses that a child with nurturing parents develops. As a result of their upbringing, these children typically don't feel "seen" by their families, and they also feel invisible in the greater world that doesn't value sensitivity. However, in all cases, empaths haven't learned to defend against stress in the same way others have.[98]"

I relate quite a bit to this description of an empath. Looking back over my life, being an empath has been confusing and the source of suffering and a fantastic ability to find common humanity and ease alienation and addictive tendencies. The practices contained herein are designed to support your process of building emotional resilience along with these other skills.

In the Singer studies[99], trainings were given to research subjects for mindfulness, empathy, and compassion. As we've discussed, the science points to experiences in different parts of the brain during compassion training and empathy training. In one study, subjects with extensive meditation experience were asked to induce empathy on demand. Those brain scans were compared with people trained in compassion meditation. They found that compassion training increased and made stronger a sense of positive emotional well-being and induced altruistic service or compassionate action for others. Some circuits related to love and

---

98 Judith Orloff. "The Empath's Survival Guide: Life Strategies for Sensitive People."

99 Tania Singer & Matthias Bolz. "Compassion - Bridging Practice and Science."

connection were enhanced. You need to know that if you're a compassionate caregiver and are experiencing compassion fatigue or empathic distress, training in the skills outlined in this book and enhancing them with additional training will lead to your increased resilience. That resilience will help you overcome the effects of being a human being constantly confronted with suffering in others.

Regulation Practice: Is it mine?

Pause in a meditation space for a few moments— Check in with how you're feeling in your body. Recall the more significant interactions of the past couple of hours. While noticing what you feel in your body, ask yourself, "Is it mine?" Consider the range of normal feelings for you in a day. Is there something that feels a bit foreign, like it doesn't belong to you, yet you still feel it? This is an important skill to develop. The ability to discern between your feelings and the feelings of others. When we notice ourselves experiencing the feelings of others, we can approach our experience with self-compassion and learn to let it go.

Option: Energetic Protection

Imagine the space around you as empty. The distance between you and anyone else's emotional experience is a buffer to have more power to choose what you let in and how much. Use your creativity to create a wand made of light for yourself. What color stands for protection for you? Some may choose red, a power color. Infuse the magic light wand with your self-compassion. Blow on it and watch the glow get bigger. Draw a circle of self-compassion around you. This will hold your space for you, just you. Nothing else will get in unless you let it. Notice how this boundary feels in your body. Allow it to help you feel more relaxed.

Empathic abilities vary among people. Some won't have much trouble; others are often exhausted because they don't know how to turn off the emotions of people around them and simply be in their own experience. Mindfulness of what you feel, and if it's yours, adds power to your practice. Just be easy with yourself. However, it is for you at the moment. Just the simple act of being aware that what you're experiencing may or may not be someone else's emotions will have a strong impact on your sense of personal agency or control, which is one of our main objectives in this guide to recovery.

Notes

Part IV

How We Recover: Principles and Practices of Compassionate Recovery

Chapter 16
Your Recovery, Your Way

"Weep not for roads untraveled
Weep not for sights unseen
May your love never end
And if you need a friend
There's a seat here alongside me[100]"
-Chester Bennington

Thank you for coming on the journey all this way! Not all of us made it. Since last night at least ten people overdosed in the USA. Five souls took their own lives. Depression and addiction are at the top of the complications due to adverse childhood experiences during crucial brain development periods. We grow up into addiction as if it's a natural course. Take one, kill the pain. Take two; kill the past. One more, and there's no tomorrow. Accumulate material wealth as if you're

---

[100] Songwriters: Brad Delson / Chester Charles Bennington / Dave Farrell / Joseph Hahn / Mike Shinoda / Robert G. Bourdon Roads Untraveled lyrics © Universal Music Publishing Group

starving to death. Reinforce the ego at a breakneck pace like you're running from the devil, but never pause long enough to notice that addiction has taken your life. Sometimes it happens quickly, sometimes slowly. The more addicted we get, the more addicted we get. Addiction is dose-related. Taking away the objects of addiction doesn't change brain chemistry. We need to be proactive.

Most people who grew up with neglected roots struggle to thrive and blossom through adulthood. According to my doctor, guys like me with an ACE of 8 should wind up pushing shopping carts downtown. This thought crosses my mind as I pass homeless, dirty, and fierce street survivors as I walk to get a slice of pizza. "The fact that you're standing here sober," she said, "is a testament to your hard work." I was in my 30s at the time.

Older now and slowing down, I feel the impact of those roots, and it's showing in my skinny branches and crumpled leaves. The work is still necessary, but it's much more challenging. Impermanence is right there, every moment.

And so is the suffering of this world if we have the heart and the capacity to notice. The measure of suffering due to these things is incomprehensible. Yet somehow, we can survive and even make our lives look good on social media.

Examples of being successful outside while dying inside are at the tip of anyone's tongue. We all know the stories. But do we know the ACE story, the addiction story, and the mental health story that underlies this? Of course not. The medical community to this day is reluctant. Therapists and other providers are coming around, but those 15 people slipped away yesterday, and 15 more will die before those efforts reach them. We need to do better, and we will do better if we live by meaning and principle. But we must be tough and beef up our capacity to cope with continuing to open up and enjoy freedom.

This material isn't easy to look at; I know that. There is a lot to take in. But like the images of war, we must not turn away from the truth if we are to understand anything about this strange and mysterious journey. We should go beyond survival into sur-thrival!

This book isn't meant to be skimmed through in an evening. Instead, everything in it is to be understood and dealt with in your time, in your own unique way. As I suggested at the beginning, keep this book with you. Share it with others. Highlight, use the notes sections. Tear out pages and tape them on the wall. Do what you need to do to make it meaningful for yourself.

If we have meaning in our life and some passion behind it, that will give us strength for the tricky parts of the journey. It's an arduous journey. Most people don't want to look at this kind of material, so we stay sick. You're looking at it. You're getting well. Dig it.

Your recovery is up to you. As my Zen teacher told me in the early 1990s, "Nobody's coming to save you." This is your moment. Each moment is a way of being. We may have been mindless, self-loathing, and uncaring of others at times in our addictions, but we're turning all of that around right now with mindfulness, self-compassion, and compassion for others.

We began the conversation with the story of ACES. Even if they don't apply to us, everything in the book applies to whatever problematic attachment-addiction you want to heal from. ACEs are an integral part of our story, my story, and children all over the world right now who are suffering what we endured and worse. They need us now, and as a society, we need to be able to serve them into adulthood. We know what the cause and effect look like in ourselves.

The impact on recovery cannot be overstated. I just got a note from a friend I've known in recovery since the mid-1980s. They have been sober for over 35 years but suffer from excruciating emotional and other problems. We were going through parts of this book, and they confided to me the specific details of their childhood, how it's impacted them all their adulthood in sobriety, and how it continues to be a struggle to this day. I learned back then, in the 80s, that there are no coincidences.

My friend who experienced the life-changing spiritual amazingness of young people in AA when it first began to share with me that the insights that I've obtained in writing this book are precisely applicable to them right now isn't a coincidence. I've known them since we were 22 years old. This was the first time I've heard the story, right in time for this book—the work we're doing here matters.

It matters to seniors in recovery because the depression and pain gets more desperate in their older years. The trauma, addiction, and trauma from addiction leave indelible scars on our deep emotional beings.

We can be mindful, bear the experience and give ourselves a new level of self-compassion. This is where healing begins, but there hasn't been a roadmap tying all of this together in a new recovery mindset, so I made one. Please use this as a tool to create your recovery roadmap.

I shared with my friend that I, too, suffer from debilitating memories. Every morning I wake up defenseless to suffering, crying out from the past. It's part of the Complex PTSD that I live with. Since I'm not alone, I wrote this book. I know that you can relate and that most readers will connect with this work. In the five years of research for this book, I spoke with several thousand people about the ideas; if you happened to be in my Uber at that time, apologies and thank you. These ideas mean nothing if they don't mean something to the people who suffer from addiction and trauma. My meaning and purpose are what I get from putting these ideas together over time in a way that intends to offer comfort and ease on the path of healing.

When I left a 30-day treatment center, the only roadmap I was given was directions to the nearest Alcoholics Anonymous group. That's the road I followed for most of my adult life. In AA, I was told to sit down, shut up, and listen. I did the opposite. I stood up, made a lot of noise, and listened to no one for several years.

One warning we often heard in meetings was that if people knew what they'd have to go through when they got sober, they wouldn't have started. But this book is telling you what you're likely to go through. Many emotional, mental, spiritual, and physical changes happen in various stages of recovery, some of which are related to trauma. General brain neuroscience gives us insight that we can use to develop further understanding. As we learn to meditate and become softer and more at ease, the wisdom of meditation reveals itself in positive and inspiring ways.

We have a basic understanding of our stress system and its role in previous traumas and current mood swings. We know something about how our brains can be reprogrammed on a neurological level through contemplative practices such as mindfulness and loving-kindness. The damage done by trauma and addiction can't be undone. But these practices get into the deep spaces where the wounds still fester. We get in there, put some kindness on it, and become a more vital, more compassionate member of our family, workplace, and community. But it takes work. We need to tolerate the reality of our condition and open our sense of self to something more comprehensive than our knots of suffering. Untie your knots. Then help somebody untie theirs. Try not to make new ones. Stay loose.

This section is about applying principles that we've been working with from the first pages. They have supported you throughout the book. Now that we have the context of how all this fits together, we can put it into a set of principles and practices for recovery that are inclusive, universal, and trauma-educated.

Rather than go into a church basement and talk about how we're addicts here. They're ordinary people out there; we leave the shame of addiction in the basement and go out in the world as a proud, shining Light of Compassion in recovery.

While this book can be used as the basis for in-person recovery groups, that's not the main point. Groups are one of many ways the work is meant to be applied. We end the isolation that kills us by integrating these practices into who we are as we interact in the world. We practice the principles from the beginning, not the end.

With all the topics we've covered, we've built a foundation of study and practice that has been good preparation for the next steps, even though there are no steps because Compassionate Recovery isn't a program that you need to follow one way. It's a way to live free. Your recovery. Your way.

We'll start with some tools for you to build a roadmap for yourself for a year. This might be your first year in recovery or your forty-third. You'll be able to select the things on your journey that you want to work on and the approaches that suit you best to work on them. You'll make a recovery meal plan from a menu that you design.

The plan is a guideline. It's fluid and dynamic in that if something's not working out according to plan, we create new neuroadaptations with something new. We don't have to pound a square peg into a round hole constantly when it's easier to craft a smoother peg more suitable to the space (of wisdom) that we're trying to enter.

Sometimes we find ourselves confused and floundering. We don't know what to do. But this is the state of mind of a panicked child. We have to remember that we're adults when it's like this. It's time to decide how we're going to be in the world. It's up to us. Put on the big gender non-specific pants and get to work.

Start Where You Are

There aren't any rules in Compassionate Recovery, so there are no excuses either. Here's the key takeaway: Wherever you are is a fine place to begin. This is true right now in this moment. It will be true tomorrow and next year. Don't know where to start? Start where you are. Don't know where you are? Check your feet. Start where you find them. In any moment of doubt and confusion, drop into your deeper wisdom right then and there. Where you are is in this moment. This moment is the right moment. Breathe in, breathe out. It's all good. The principles act as natural laws that don't need to be reinforced.

You have a very low tolerance for your own excuses. With everything we've learned so far, before you read on, what do you think the core problem is if you find yourself in a situation where you feel overwhelmed, baffled, and confused?

If you said dysregulation, that is correct. When you don't eat all day, executive function suffers. We wouldn't show up to a job interview after staying up all night[101]. Regulation of our circuitries will ground us to get some clarity. So, if you're confused, grounding is your move. This is an example of the application of our study.

As children, we had no idea what was happening to our systems. Now we have technology, research, and experience to provide a framework for seeing ourselves in a new light. Our self-reference or view of ourselves changes for the better when we apply this knowledge. Knowledge must be practical, or it's just words.

---

[101] Anymore.

We need to regulate and write a new narrative of who we are and aspire to be. That being the goal, we have the destination. Now we look at what is required to get there. After that, we look at the year, month, week, or day and ask what steps we need to take to get there? This process is the same for any project. The objective defines the path. Our objective in recovery is to feel great and do well. Getting there involves steps. You will need to keep your goals attainable. Set yourself up for success. Don't set a trap that will put you in a spiral where you feel you've failed. You define the objective and the rate at which you'll work to get there. It's like planning a trip. When you get to this destination, you'll arrive with new mood dynamics, better physical health, more robust coping mechanisms, and a brighter smile. Just think of how great the pictures will be!

Make a Roadmap

If you've ever snow skied, you know how to pick your path down the mountain. If you want to have fun, maybe you'll hit some moguls. If it's early morning and the fresh powder is untracked while snowflakes are falling, take a slower run to enjoy the scenery. In your recovery, you're the skier. Pick a fall line, then shred it up. Consider where you're going and how we want to feel when we get there.

The principle applies to non-skiers, don't worry. Defining your path gives a structure or a way to hold space for yourself and your energy. When you give your world structure, energy knows where it can flow and where the edges are. When you make this structure for yourself, you guide yourself, your energy, through a path.

I discovered this when making mindful Zen harmony pathways around my longer-term camper spots. Pathways are cool to look at and an excellent way to have a wellness practice in your yard if you have the space. Buy the monks walk mindfully, feeling or even blessing the Earth with every movement of every step. If there's another monk in front of us, we don't walk to push them. Everyone is responsible for keeping up with the person in front of them, one step at a time.

The idea of a roadmap is super simple. You can use something as simple as Google Calendar on your phone to set Goals. This idea is to first make some goals and plans for your recovery with the help of your team, then put commitments on digital paper. Make a schedule that you can and will do. It's not a regimen but a flexible, dynamic path. You won't be able to predict what happens ahead, but you'll have a plan and account for contingencies.

A word about structure: wear it like a loose shirt. In other words, don't trip. Structure can go too far. Don't let it.

In early recovery, your life needs to be very structured, so your roadmap for the year will look different than someone further along. Your issues will include fundamental stability issues such as housing, resolving legal issues, employment, financial and credit status, childcare, and custody. Someone with 37 years of sobriety who's suffering from excruciating complex PTSD with a life that looks otherwise perfect will need to solve other problems with different tools.

No one roadmap is right for everyone, just like there's not one pill that cures all illnesses. For this reason, we need a way to choose our adventure. There are many ways to do this, including mind maps, legal pads, and dry erase boards. Choose your tool. For simplicity, I'll use a spreadsheet as an example. In the first column, you'll list the things you'd like to work on. This is totally unique to your recovery journey, and you'll find people to support and share the experience with. The second column is for healing tools, activities, or anything that supports your well-being and addresses the specifics you deem important.

For the issues in column one, break out each issue into physical, mental, emotional, and spiritual categories. If your issue is toxic relationships, list out some things to work on in the physical category first. What can you address to compassionately feed your health and soul? Think of fun things that involve movements, such as a dance class or mindful walking. In terms of emotions, list a few problems for you, such as anxiety, depression, or sadness.

You're only going to work on one thing at a time, but you'll put more stuff on the list as you go. Don't freak out about how many things there are to work on. When we work with a mindful, compassionate intention on our brains, the healing will affect more than one area. All the principles and practices in Compassionate Recovery work together to support you and the wider community. This is an example of organizing your thoughts to make a plan that will help you work on aspects of yourself that you and your circle of support/safety decide are important and doable in your recovery, whatever that may be.

You can do this. However, it works best for you. List out the areas to work on in no particular order. Just brainstorm. Then seek solutions and list those. You will draw from these and put them into a calendar of action items that you will commit to practicing consistently.

Break everything down into the four components of your reality. Take care of all of them in the specific ways that are needed. For example, what will you do to protect and strengthen your emotional stability? Add tools like therapy, support groups, and yoga classes. Mentally, what do you want to study to fill the gaps? List some books, courses, or workshops that could help. On the spiritual dimension, how can you apply some tools from your spiritual toolkit? We have plenty to choose from that work in a secular and a spiritual manner, such as mindfulness.

Things to work on	Ways it affects me	Priorities
effects of a toxic relationship:		
Physically	Exhaustion, lack of appetite, tremors	Physical safety, restraining order, move, change number. Prepare a go-bag with cash, ID, and an extra phone and car keys.
Mentally	Unable to focus, out of the window of tolerance on the low side	Communicate with support team, outpatient group regularly
Emotionally	Numb	Do self-compassion practices 3x daily
Spiritually	Empty	Spend time in nature

Ask yourself the questions that you need answers to. If you put it out there, answers will come from surprising places.

What is your short-, medium- and long-term destination? Is it to be comfortable in your own skin, find a mate that won't hurt you, or get an online certification?

Where do you want to be in one year regarding your physical, emotional, mental, and spiritual wellbeing? Do you want to be a better parent, a more effective communicator, or a helpful neighbor?

What kind of emotional everyday feeling state would you like to develop over the next year? What would it feel like?

Is there someone that you would like to emulate that expresses this feeling, a song, perhaps? Try writing one.

What color or color set makes you feel like you've already arrived at this healthier place? Get a hat or tattoo in those colors, but don't tell anyone why.

If we make a meal plan, we need a recipe and ingredients. You may need to research the kinds of studies and activities that will suit your feeling about how you want to develop yourself. When I was in my 20s in early recovery, my favorite things to do were personal development and spiritual workshops. I love engaging with interesting people, whether they are in sales training or a spiritual master. Looking back over time, I can see that this is the passion I should have been spending time on instead of sitting in smoke-filled rooms of 12-step meetings. But we were conditioned to be so afraid that if we didn't stick close to the program, we would drink. I wound up doing many years of personal, educational, and spiritual development.

For this reason, I encourage you to do more fun things that will make your life better and worry less. Don't be lazy and fall into a funnel trap. If your goal is recovery, do what you have to do. You must want it. Nobody can do that for you. But if you don't know that, at least know that you're sick of the way your life has been going, and you want to do the deep healing work.

If you're already a very organized and structured person, plug compassionate, mindful recovery activities into your existing routine. Otherwise, here are some examples of how you could map out a day, a week, a month, and a year of recovery plans to guide you.

Start with bigger goals and work your way down as you place the menu items onto your calendar or into a planner.

2023 Sample Recovery Roadmap

Compassion Training	Complete online course in social media
Internal Family Systems Therapy	Read five books on spirituality
Marial arts classes	Study Non-violent Communication
Art therapy	Form a community group to save stray pets
Rock climbing	Enter a stand-up open mic

These are a few of the unlimited number of recovery-positive things to do. There is no limit to how creative you can be or how much fun you can make your life in recovery. It's important for self-regulation, mindful living, and recovery development. We can and should plan to improve and grow. Put it on paper and make commitments. If you do recovery planning for a year, you will be stunned at the changes you'll see manifest in your life.

Part of making a roadmap is knowing where the obstacles in the road might be. We may or may not need chains, but we'll wish we had them if it snows. It's best to be prepared to avoid unnecessary detours and breakdowns. We can never plan for everything, but when we plan, we feel regulated, less confused, and our lives become un-chaotic, even boring[102].

Integration Practice: Annual Recovery Plan

Do this annually or biannually. Get together with some people in recovery once a week for four weeks. It can be at any time of the year. Choose a team leader who will be responsible for coordinating the sessions. Get together first to brainstorm the things that you need to work on. If you do this alone, it's not as fun, and you'll miss out on getting super emo with your friends and having them pull your covers about what needs work. The second session will be about creating a menu of healing tools, life-affirming activities, and anything that your group can come up with that addresses the particular issues you discovered, processed, and journaled on from the week before—Journal between meetups. The third session will be for committing to the plan.

In this session, the group creates a ritual for celebrating the coming together, sharing of common humanity, and supporting each other in the ongoing, dynamic phase of recovery that you find yourselves in at that moment. Make it a party, make it a game, go to the Farmer's Market, or a nature walk. Light candles, sit, and sob. Burn old

---

102 If we're lucky.

resentments on paper in a safe firepit in the backyard. Say a prayer together, make an earth mandala, and go to a concert of music you've never heard before.

Your recovery, your way.

Notes

Chapter 17
Funnel Traps

"Play every note as if it's your last."
-Flea

To make it in recovery, we can't give up. It takes strong effort and consistency. Recovery also requires flexibility in what we do, think, feel, *and* are empowered by. These principles will take us a long way on the path of recovery. Conversely, our dedication to the principles of laziness, flakiness, and rigidity cause nothing but misery. We cannot foresee everything. Shit will go wrong. So, when you get caught off guard and find yourself in a funnel trap, it's important to have backup plans in your phone, ready to be implemented with people who know what to expect and have agreed to support you.

Make plans, but don't be attached to everything working out as you expect. We learn and grow on the path. It's unnecessary to craft the perfect recovery plan, especially if you're new to it. The act of thinking about it at all will put you miles ahead. That said, some unexpected topics are likely to come up on your road of recovery. This chapter offers a few more flares to steer you around trouble. May they light your way and help avoid potholes.

Get started on a list of ideas for contingencies that might trip you up and land you in the funnel. Set up a journal for such funnel traps. With your team, write the action plan. The plan in your pocket will say who to call if you wind up in a state of distress or feel it coming on. Learn to monitor your ups and downs, then take them to your peer group for discussion. Do consistent check-ins. Be prepared for contingencies on the road of compassion.

How do you know what can happen? You know from looking at the past patterns through your recovery work. It'd be good to get at it if that's all mystery to you because progress takes time and work. It's all hard. But you're doing it. You can pause and make a conscious choice to be joyous about that.

Many things will reveal themselves on their own, but some of the deep issues in our tissues can be pretty stubborn. If the work just came naturally, we wouldn't need any help. This stuff is hard because it's hard. It's buried for a reason. The toxic stress from allostatic overload that continues on a chronic basis without hope for escape digs deep neuro grooves into our circuits.

It's buried for survival. This locked-in trauma energy can be profound. To experience it all at once would be too much for our system. The material will come up with mindfulness training and compassion training. On the journey, as we utilize these concepts of a multifaceted, comprehensive approach to recovery, our work will present itself to us. Be ready for some of the possible contingencies, which will jumpstart your neural network to build a new knowledge base of healing possibilities.

I've struggled with the epiphany that my life has definite patterns every many years. These are things that I can now trace back to childhood and later years. Bipolar things. Addiction things and trauma things. We all have patterns and, as we discussed, spirals that intertwine and go up and down. But you don't see what you're in when you're in it. If you don't want the truth, you know how to avoid it. I know I sure did.

This crash and burn pattern was probably obvious to everybody else but me. But it's now useful information for my health and wellbeing. For example, if I want to know the patterns in a future relationship, I can go through the things that I've done selfishly in the past as predictors. But those predictors can be chanced with conscious intention.

Those are things we naturally tend to avoid, but the value of looking squarely at and checking in on your patterns is that you can protect yourself, prevent old patterns and try new approaches. One such pattern that we need to change is this feeling that we are diseased and broken.

Am I Diseased?

There may be no way around the norm of referring to addicts as having a disease, which we do, but that's not the problem. The problem is that we over-identify with it and ourselves as flawed.

In the treatment field, there is debate on whether it's a good idea to call addiction a disease. There is a movement away from using this label because it's overly stigmatizing. I've called it a disease since 1984. Although I have criticisms of different aspects of the treatment field, I've personally never questioned the idea of addiction being a disease.

"disease noun

dis·ease | \ di-ˈzēz \

Definition of disease

1: a condition of the living animal or plant body or of one of its parts that impairs normal functioning and is typically manifested by distinguishing signs and symptoms: SICKNESS, MALADY.[103]"

If you look at this definition, it's hard to understand why people write whole books and articles arguing against calling addiction a disease. Addiction is a condition. It's easy to see it as a condition that impairs normal functioning. Anyone who's been an addict or been affected by addiction knows that it impairs normal functioning in about

---

[103] https://www.merriam-webster.com/dictionary/disease

two and a half seconds. There is extensive, well-validated brain research that makes it abundantly clear. But we don't have to blame "our disease" for everything. It's an overgeneralization.

As we've seen, there are likely numerous health issues that we're likely to have due to ACEs. Addiction is part of that list, but it doesn't define us. The more language that we use to make it define us, the more we push ourselves into a shame-based sense of alienation. It's better to be OK with the disease aspect, since it's reality, and let it go. Identify with self-compassion instead.

Compassionate Recovery doesn't insist that you call addiction a disease or do *not* call it a disease. All points are valid, even if we disagree. Well, especially if we disagree.

If we use our sliding scale definition of a spectrum of addiction that begins with unhealthy attachment and moves to full-blown addiction in the end, then it doesn't matter if you think of addiction as a disease or not. It only matters if you understand that you have a problem and need a solution. If you continue to use dangerous drugs while trying to figure out your position on addiction as a disease, you may die trying. Let's not have that.

You Are Not Broken

Hello, my name is Darren. I am compassionate.

To practice self-compassion in recovery, choose positive identifiers that foster self-empowerment. We often identify as broken, wounded, powerless addicts. Every time we say it, we hear ourselves, and it gets imprinted. We may be powerless over an addiction, but most of us superimpose that on other aspects of ourselves, which is not fair to those parts of ourselves.

Just imagine if the part of you that feels empowered were sitting next to the part of you, that feels powerless. What would they say to each other? Begin a writing process using this technique with different aspects of yourself.

A word that embodies loving-kindness would be a supportive identifier to use. Every time we hear ourselves say it, it gets imprinted. We could say, "Hello, my name is Andy. I am Aware." Based on this identification, people could share what they're aware of in their addiction-recovery process. It might look something like,

I'm Andy, and I am aware. I'm aware of my desire to not drink or use today. I'm aware of the discomfort in my body due to anger from a situation that happened at work.

It's important to our recovery, especially if we're at the severely addicted end of the spectrum, to never forget where we came from. But there's a way to do that without re-traumatizing ourselves. We can reframe the way we speak about our addictions. This will impact how we feel and what we do:

I remember what it was like when I was using.

When I was active in my addiction, I had no control over the amount I would take.

Addiction brought me to my knees and left me in a state of absolute powerlessness to control it.

We can use any positive identifier that we want. We just want to choose identifiers that support growth and wellness and a positive, compassionate way of speaking about ourselves and each other. Use this or create your own list.

My name is _____, and

- I am kind
- I am self-empowered
- I am compassionate
- I'm OK in my own skin
- I'm working on my attachments
- I'm working on my addictions
- I am loving
- I have a good heart
- I am forgiving
- I'm strong
- I am joyous
- I am free
- I am present

Remember, these are identifiers and affirmations. You're drawing on these energies and building a neural but also an emotional-energetic network of lovingkindness within yourself. To identify is to become one with. Live it. Like the method actor, step into it, become it. Feel it. Be it. This powerful shift in mindset will alter everything if applied sincerely. I've been working on it since the 1980s. It works.

What would your hero do? What would it be like if you were your hero? What would it look like, feel like, taste like? In this case, you're repurposing the part of your brain[104] where your sense of self resides to a powerful, compassionate new programmable memory.

What if you feel crapola and aren't in the mood for positive thinking? Rather than say things that we don't feel, we try to start where we are. This is an excellent practice and permits us to be who we are and when we are. Instead of saying, "I'm JoAnne, and I'm depressed," identify with the solution. Say, "I'm JoAnne, and my feet are on the floor. I'm in my body. A little on the low end of my window of tolerance."

Acknowledge how you feel without over-identifying with the problem because how we feel is not the whole truth of our entire being. It's a part of our humanity, but we are complex. That part is not the entire story.

I might feel broken. Sad. Sick. Powerless. But the feelings, trauma, and addiction history don't have to define me. I can choose. There is new awareness on my skin. The sounds coming to me are myriad. There is so much going on in the space around me, even if it needs a closer look.

Start where you are, the new present moment awareness. As you progress, move into realizing the potential of being your most evolved, happiest self.

We get to choose how we want to define ourselves. The words carry vibrations that heal those

---

104 Do you remember which part?

of deep shame. The identifier we use has an important effect on how we feel; we must remember that we still need to. We choose to live a life of self-compassion and compassion for others. That runs opposite to how we act amid addictions. The identifier is an important step toward deeper self-compassion and mindful, present moment, non-judgmental awareness. It's a beginning on the path, not the end result. We change our narrative, a vital front-line therapeutic tool in the trauma field. You can get support for this.

This kind of rewrite helps guide our emotional state and frees up space to act with upgraded words and deeds that teach us to feel safe in our space. The more regulated we get, the more regulated we get. Self-regulation is dose-related.

Inflation

The flip side of identifying as less than is to identify as more than you really are. You may be able to know out one hell of an "I Will Always Love You" at the karaoke bar, but that doesn't make you Whitney! If you do think you're Whitney, that's inflation.

The legendary Swiss Psychoanalyst C.G. Jung[105] is who first called this phenomenon inflation. When

---

[105] Schlamm L. (2014) Inflation. In: Leeming D.A. (eds) Encyclopedia of Psychology and Religion. Springer, Boston, MA. https://doi.org/10.1007/978-1-4614-6086-2_330 For a deeper

we join a spiritually inspiring group, we tend to over-identify with the group. Sometimes people in recovery can over-identify with their higher power or the divine inspiration of the AA literature. The erroneous conclusion that some come to is that because they've studied followed the instructions, and memorized the one and only sacred book, they are the message when they're just a messenger. Being able to stay sober despite lousy behavior doesn't make us legit. In fact, this is a kind of faux legitimacy.

Inflation can also be called spiritual pride, but inflation can go further. When it does go wild, people can do some crazy things. Think about how right-wing nationalist groups and other cults work. Sports teams count on inflation or over-identification with the team as rivals brawl it out in the parking lot. What happens is that we expand our personality into something beyond ourselves.

It can be a religious figure, or we may feel that we're channeling Jimi Hendrix. There's no reason to suggest that channeling isn't authentic because many people channel. But when we start to think that we are the super cool thing we're identifying with, the trouble begins.

This happens a lot in yoga and meditation communities. As a yoga teacher for many years, I

---

examination of inflation and Tibetan deity yoga, see Hopkins, Jeffrey. "Jung's Warnings Against Inflation." Chung-hwa Buddhist Journal 21 (2008): 159-174.

can admit that, at times, I felt that I was the important factor in the equation. But a real yogi knows that the only way to channel the good energy is to let the ego step aside. If our ego identity is more important than the flow of the teaching, it's pretty lame and obvious to everybody except the inflated teacher. I've done it. We all do it. Don't do it.

You need to know that inflation is a yellow blinking light on the road to expanding our self-definition and connecting to a larger sense of community that is, ultimately, without limits. It's very seductive for the ego to tell us, "Yeah, that's all about you, baby. You got the juice!" But it's somebody or something else's, or, as Jung believed, we even identify with something we make up. In fact, the nobody else's juice.

We will be pumped up to be part of something bigger than us, which is one of the main points of this book. But when it becomes more important than compassion, remember it's just you. Inflation is a funnel trap for people recovering from addictions because we superimpose our addiction-starved ego onto anything that will cover up our sense of personal inadequacy. This isn't a slam on low self-esteem, but it is a red flag. Inflation, says Jung, is a coverup. The ego without its addictions can go on rampages of bloated self-importance because we belong to some special club, race, belief system, or sexual identity, be it real or imagined. In Compassionate Recovery, the club is the planet you're sitting on right now[106]. We are all in the same boat. Knowing that and acting on it applies the principle of common humanity. It's pretty tasty medicine for the parts of us that are raw and needs some self-compassion.

To avoid inflation, as we expand ourselves into bigger and healthier things, we need to develop discernment through mindfulness. But mindfulness can also be inflation. We over-identify with being the mindful one. Checking mindfulness will awaken the circuits we discussed earlier that give us clarity and insight. It's like flipping a switch, as we've done throughout the book.

We need a pit-stop on the road to mastery, be it proficiency in a personal, interpersonal, professional, or spiritual skill. In this view, we take the approach of limitless possibility rather than sad brokenness. In that regard, some humility about the ego's insatiable urge to inflate itself is helpful to us in our practice of compassion. But without road checks from our circle of safety pit crew, some of this might go unchecked.

We should consistently seek the honest evaluation of our circle of safety, which should always include a licensed clinician educated in these matters. If your therapist isn't educated in this area, please show them your copy of this book. It's important to use clinicians who are properly

---

106 Unless you read while walking, in which case please make that adjustment.

knowledgeable about these issues to make appropriate choices for our health and well-being.

This is like what we learned about empathy. There's a point where we must be able to discern the other person's distress from our own experience, or we'll spiral out of tolerance ourselves. We need to know who we are and who we are not. We can find out more about who we are by not being who we aren't. Be careful of inflation. Here are some warning signs.

If you feel that you know the truth and nobody else does.

If you feel like a god.

If you feel like a demon.

The force of the inflation can bring us to a place where we might think we're more human than human. Check it. Then have it checked. Compassion is a higher principle that takes us to a level of conscious awareness beyond ourselves, which is great if we don't fall into the trap that our compassion is better—or worse than anyone else's. Remember, inflation works both ways.

Spiritual Bypassing

Whether our endeavors are on the physical, mental, emotional, or spiritual planes, if we inflate our understanding before it's ripe, we're liable to miss the natural sweetness of the fruit. We think we know, but we don't know what we don't know. It would be as if we were going to New York City from San Diego and stopped off in Albuquerque at a New York Pizza and called it good. In Compassionate Recovery, you're not required to be spiritual or secular or care about either. But there is an intense and powerful non-material something going on when it comes to the healing power of compassion.

If we go to a recovery group, meditation, or self-compassion course and come home preaching for the family, we will have missed, sidestepped, or bypassed the point. The point is the work, and work is the point. It's about our own work. If people want what we have, they'll ask. It's compassionate to respect people's boundaries.

A psychologist and Buddhist practitioner, John Wellwood, coined the term spiritual bypassing over thirty years ago. It happens when we use spiritual, healing, empowering practices, and affiliations to avoid facing our wounds. Because most spiritual, recovery, and similar groups aren't utilizing the big picture, there are blind spots that people fall into. This shouldn't happen with those following this book because, for one thing, we're talking about it up front instead of not knowing or not wanting to know that it exists.

In short, a spiritual bypasser thinks they're more spiritual than they are. Wellwood says that bypassers think they've transcended when they're still on the ground.

Robert Augustus Masters, author of *Spiritual Bypassing,* holds that we confuse surface with depth in spiritual bypassing. When we first start practicing a new path, it's easy to get excited, but we're skimming the surface until we do some study and practice and have enough time to go through what life brings us.

Bypassing happens when we first get into recovery and have a moment of clarity. We convince ourselves that we've found something valuable, so we run around spreading the gospel to our addict friends, which always works out great, right?

When we're in the know-it-all headspace, we really don't know shite. Funnel traps like this are tricky. When we realize we're in it, all we can hear is the flush. Best keep our eyes on the road until we get where we're going.

Surrender

Surrender to compassion. Compassion can be seen as spiritual, as it is the basis of all spiritual systems. It bears repeating that compassion can be thought of as a secular practice for those not comfortable with spirituality. Either way, we look at it, the practice of compassion is the deepest practice that we humans can do if we surrender to it.

The notion of letting go of an attachment is like surrendering our grip on it, hence the term. The more we hold on, the less we surrender. This resistance is a funnel trap because it's an ace in the hole for us if we decide to go back into addiction. Letting go means letting go. It's an absolute surrender if you want it to work.

Remember, in this approach; we're about fluidity rather than rigidity. Be relaxed and flexible. Adapt to change. Give up the fight. It's commonly said in recovery that we surrender to win. But for the traumatized, the notion of surrender can be a trigger unless we surrender to self-compassion.

We learn to let the ego dissolve through self-compassion rather than an attitude of force. They talk about puncturing the ego and smashing our delusions in recovery communities, but Compassionate Recovery takes a softer approach. It's kind of like sitting in the dentist's chair. You know it will hurt, but you just have to relax and get through it. Then you walk out with a great new smile. As I was finishing this book, I had six root canals. There was nothing to do but surrender. Since I get to eat normal food, I win.

Instead of surrendering to some authority or set of rules, we choose to surrender our fear, anxiety, and anger to the practice of self-compassion and compassion for others. Through the practices in this book, we learn to surrender gently and land more softly. This eases the shock wave that we have on others too.

Practice:
Surrender to Compassion

To get a feeling for soft surrender, try this simple practice. Find a spot you can chill for a few minutes.

Become still.

Become silent.

Become aware.

Whatever you're doing, just pause and notice your condition. Observe your thoughts without following them. Notice any resistance. Notice the desire, need, or even the compulsion to fix yourself. If the feelings are strong, just notice the physical sensation and let the moment be.

Let every aspect of your experience be exactly as it is in this moment. Be compassionate to yourself by relaxing any pressure to be anything other than who you are in this moment, without changing a thing.

That's a soft surrender. Let yourself linger there.

Return to this practice often. It's dose-related.

Like all the practices in Compassionate Recovery, these get better, deeper, stronger, and more fun over time. The good news is that you're in charge of what you practice and when. Look at the following resource for some excellent ideas on making a roadmap. Even if you don't identify with mental illness, identify with mental health.

The National Alliance for Mental Illness, or NAMI, is a national resource center for mental health education, advocacy, and support. It was founded in 1977 by Harriet Shetler and Beverly Young, who both had children diagnosed with schizophrenia. Their core values are hope, the inclusion of everybody, self-empowerment, and compassion. One of their programs is a Wellness Recovery Action Plan or WRAP[107].

Sobriety First

We can't get into recovery until we achieve abstinence from our addictions. If we're in harm reduction, that's a different deal. But for those who aren't in that severe of a situation, we begin recovery with abstinence from the abuser. No texting, obsessing, driving by, social media stalking…you know the drill. The drug is the drug is the drug. It doesn't matter what it is, as we have fully established. If you're still in active addictions, get into treatment. Take this book with you to keep you company. But you need to get off the crack to get into some healing.

There are stages of change regarding getting to the point where you get sober. First, you become aware of the problem, then we think about it for a while, do some research maybe. Eventually, we start looking for help. Sometimes we get help. Maybe we even make some changes. Ultimately, we get serious

---

[107] https://www.wellnessrecoveryactionplan.com

and do the real work. That's what Compassionate Recovery is about.

Length of sobriety on one particular addiction does not equate to a mindful, compassionate lifestyle. We need to be abstinent and do the work.

How Much Time You Got?

Recovery can't be measured by time, but sobriety must. While it's true that recovery is just for today, it's also about a lot of today's in a row if we want to make progress. In Compassionate Recovery, however, we go for quality over quantity. Days of continuous sobriety are required for successful brain healing. That's an indisputable fact. If you want to keep playing around with your addictions, you won't get far on your recovery-mastery path.

The amount of time sober can be used as a faux qualifier for qualities that we'd like to develop, such as generosity, patience, a great work ethic, and the pursuit of knowledge. We can bear down and help others 24/7 and stay sober ourselves and never touch one of these issues nor develop these qualities. So, while it's about time in some ways, namely that we need not interrupt our healing with relapses, it's not really about time. For that reason, rather than focus on days, months, and years sober, we'll put our mindful, compassionate attention on the qualities that we want to develop and aspire to.

The reality is that addicts can get a coin for five years off alcohol but have zero recovery on sex addiction, smoking, or gambling. To focus on the time is to miss the point. It's about what we do with the time, not the days on the calendar. But that is not an excuse to forget about days on the calendar. That's a nuance that we must understand.

Time is necessary but not sufficient.

In the decades that I've been in recovery, I've often felt even though I wasn't drinking or using; I wasn't well on other dimensions. I felt broken in many areas, such as relationships, finances, and most importantly, emotional stability. My definition of recovery had to expand. Once it did, a lot of knots started to loosen.

Compassionate Recovery is open and inclusive to all levels and types of attachments and addictions. One clean date for one addiction is important to note, but it's not the focus, just as meetings in church basements are fine as part of our recovery if that's what we want to participate in, but it's not the main focus.

It must be this way, and it works out well because we're not dealing with one substance or behavior in this approach. We're looking at an overall tendency toward attachment-addiction, and a comprehensive approach to recovery that leads to mastery; personal, professional, creative, educational, or spiritual.

Instead of a 30-day token for not using oxycontin, we can carry Compassion Coins with aspirations of our roadmaps to compassion and mastery. These will be available at compassioanterecovery.us soon. Remember, every moment counts.

Emotional Sobriety

Speaking of recovery that can't be measured in days and weeks, we wouldn't be able to say that we had something like abstinence from emotional addiction with any credibility unless we monitored our emotions daily with sophisticated measures. [108]But with what we know about the brain, it's clear that emotions can be addictive, especially those related to stress. We get jacked up on getting jacked up. And the more jacked up we get, the more jacked up we get. It's dose-related. We can become drama junkies, bored if things are quiet and stable. Can you relate to that? If you can, you're like me. Emotional sobriety isn't talked about that much, but emotional self-regulation is key to living a mindful, self-compassionate life in recovery. When we learn to stop getting high on emotional intensity and drama, we begin to live in an emotionally sober way.

It is challenging to retool our innate emotional responses, particularly considering childhood

---

108 Maybe one day we'll have an emotional Fitbit where that can be possible.

intensity and the vicissitudes of life in active addiction. With our core principles of mindfulness and compassion, we can slowly but surely progress towards a life where we don't actively seek out the drama. We learn to be OK with a life that looks boring by the standards of active addiction in all its glory. We become comfortable in our own skin and can create an empathic resonance with others that helps them feel stable and grounded as well. As a stress junkie, I've had to actively learn to stop myself from creating stress where there is none. Emotional sobriety is a day-by-day process with many ups and downs. If I lose my shit and start screaming in traffic, I'll have to be honest and call that an emotional relapse. When I argue with an ex that I shouldn't be talking to anyway, I need to reevaluate my commitment to my emotional sobriety.

This is where the good ole bread and butter values of honesty, integrity, and diligence come in handy. But we apply them to ourselves, with the help of our recovery community, including everyone, because we're in the world together, supporting each other with empathy and compassion.

It's good to surround ourselves with calm, compassionate, stable people to learn to use our mirror neurons and intentional self-compassion practices to rebuild our sense of emotional presence. At some point, we allow beauty and joy to arise and let pass the aches and tears. This is a state of equanimity that reflects the ancient seers' teachings. It can be done, it is being done. You need to know that you can do it, and the good news is you don't have to do it alone.

Remember, we can be sober from substances, yet not sober from emotional intoxication due to our dysregulations. Ergo, it is useful for us and our energy to be mindful, self-compassionate, and considerate to ourselves and others.

Psychedelic Sobriety

Plant medicine is healing when we're ready for it. When you're ready is up to you. If you're on narcotics or are deep into alcoholism, I wouldn't do any of this work without several years of abstinence and therapy under my belt. Some disagree. It's up to you. If you think you're going to bring a freaked-out addict mind into a hard-core psychedelic journey, good luck. I've made these journeys extensively. We must have some stability and ability to regulate before exposing ourselves to work that could kill us if we're not ready.

Many people also use small micro doses of different things that some may not consider total abstinence in the treatment world. This is a popular and hot topic not only in recovery but elsewhere. I've met many who use different substances such as Ibogaine, DMT, LSD, THC, MDMA, and psilocybin *to treat, not cause* addiction.

Things that we could in the past take and consider ourselves in relapse are now being used to initiate and sustain recovery. This is revolutionary. And it's not just a bunch of hippie weirdos. Trained, educated, intelligent people are doing this work[109]. Treatments for anxiety, depression, and addiction are being developed right now.

We'll have to deal with this in another volume. This whole area is exploding and will be a hot topic in the recovery field going forward. If you're interested, tell Google to send you articles with the keywords to your phone or device. A lot is happening nationwide.

Some recovery groups are forming that are interested in this path. What's missing is a recovery group that is stable, with long-term sobriety from their main drugs of choice, with experience going through life's hurdles sober, and has experience and interest in the long-term benefits of using these medicines as part of the healing process and not some bullshit excuse to use.

The use of these has everything to do with the intention behind it. Are you trying to catch a buzz, escape your feelings, or otherwise avoid reality? Or are you trying to heal? This is a sensitive area. To navigate it requires some skill. That there is a

---

[109] Psychedelics as Medicines: An Emerging New Paradigm. Nichols, Johnson, Nichols 2017

movement is undeniable. It's happening, whether we agree on it or not. What would happen if we approached plant medicine with the principles contained in this book?

The basic principle of recovery is that if you're high on something, then you're not sober. If you want to be sober, you don't take things that get you high. But people and situations are complicated, and there are grey areas. Medication-Assisted Treatment or MAT uses drug agents and psychotherapy to facilitate abstinence from opiates and other substances. There are clinicians currently using psychotropic medications for all kinds of emotional problems. These can have side effects, however.

Much of the science on why they work is vague and controversial. While I encourage people in recovery to consider the medical community's advice, it's also important to do actual, legit research and be a good consumer of these services. Always use a qualified, reputable guide that has good ratings.

Supersize Your McMindfulness[110]

In 1991, I was at Cal State Long Beach studying Psychology while working on my spiritual program

---

[110] McMindfulness: How Mindfulness Became the New Capitalist Spirituality 2019 Ronald Purser

along the way. I was doing both because my idea was to be a spiritually oriented psychologist, which was almost unheard of. If you had mentioned mindfulness, nobody would have known what you were talking about back then. Things have changed. Where once we had to go to India to find a meditation retreat, now the employees of Space X can go to mindfulness and ayahuasca weekends with their bosses.

Most therapists and yoga teachers who think they're therapists teach mindfulness. You can even get certified as a genuine mindfulness teacher, certified by a guy who went to a weekend workshop and started a business from it.

Trauma is a common language in TV and movies, and if you had any questions about what it's like to be a Single Drunk Female, there isn't much left unsaid. Practices like mindfulness and yoga were in the fringe back in the day. Though our yuppie friends thought we were weird, there was respect for these Eastern traditions. Things have changed.

This trend of integrating principles like mindfulness into the mainstream isn't a bad thing. But if we lose the connection to where it comes from, it's not going to work very well in the long run, beyond some basic benefits. Mindfulness is and has always been a tool to take you into your deepest reality. Don't sell yourself short by hooking up with a sellout marketing program that's more hype than hardcore.

We need the real deal, not the corporate rebranded version, when it comes to our recovery and well-being. Each moment, as it is, belongs to us and can't be bought or sold. McMindfulness in a bottle may be on the shelf soon, but it will be empty of wisdom calories.

According to a keyword search, we can find books on

- Neoliberal mindfulness
- The mantra of stress
- Privatizing mindfulness
- Mindfulness as social amnesia
- Mindfulness' truthiness problem
- Mindful employees
- Mindful merchants
- Mindful elites
- Mindful schools
- Mindful warriors
- Mindful politics

The idea that mindfulness programs will increase productivity is born out in the research, as are the studies on empathy and compassion training as economically beneficial to the company's bottom line.

The mindfulness practices in this book are intended to steer you deeper on your road. Of course, we want to be mindful of McMindful-esque teachers and programs. But what we need to be mindful of is this co-opting of mindfulness by the ego, which makes a big project out of it. Instead of being raw and humble and truthful, our practice is a commodity that we can trade to make the ego feel important and knowledgeable. It's a trap.

We don't get something from mindfulness. However, if we practiced it with our whole being, we would be surrendering completely. If we corporatize what our most important inner work, our CEO, the ego will come up with all kinds of ways to make the practice anything but what it is actually about. If that sounds like you, don't worry. We all do it. The practice is catching and releasing. We become aware that we're distracted and release that distraction. Return to mindfulness practice.

That's how we don't sell out to the man.

Mindfulness, yoga, compassion, tattoos, and being a rebel Buddhist were all things that were hipster, underground, or even outlaw, like riding a Harley Davidson motorcycle. But nowadays, the nerdiest people have full sleeve tattoos; corporations run the multibillion-dollar yoga business, and doctors ride Harleys. This doesn't mean that Harleys are any less quality or that yoga is less beneficial than before corporate America monopolized all of these things. It just means that to find the true value in the practices, we need to do the real work. McMindfulness is just another form of spiritual bypassing.

Mindfulness alone can lead to issues. I remember sitting in the Zen center on retreats and feeling like a live wire. Trauma comes to the surface for those who sit still long enough to let it. But the deeper you go, the deeper you go. Learning to meditate and handle what comes up takes a long time. It also takes context and support.

We need to be aware that the true depth of these practices and their real benefit comes from taking them seriously, getting very honest with ourselves, and trusting those in our support system to tell us the truth as they see it. Mindfulness and compassion are skills that need to be sharpened and honed over time.

There are a couple of things to watch out for when we practice real mindfulness and integrated self-compassion. One is excitement. The other is fatigue. These two are obstacles to clarity. In the window of tolerance, we know that there's a space where we can exist comfortably until something triggers us and become too excited or too fatigued. Mindfulness practices can help us immensely with knowing where we are in our window of tolerance to regulate ourselves. This is a significant improvement over not knowing what's happening and falling victim to addictive impulses.

Practice: Want some tempeh fries with that?

Sit in your meditation position. Decide what you're going to be mindful of. In this case, we'll choose the rising and falling of the belly as you breathe. Decide that you're going to focus on this and not forget. Make that commitment for 10 minutes. Of course, you will forget to focus on your belly, probably sooner than later. Then what? Vigilance is keeping a watchful eye on your mindfulness practice. When you forget, come back to the object of meditation.

When we realize we become distracted, we don't follow the idea or sensation. Instead, we come back to the object of our focus. That's the practice. There's a part of us that remembers and a part of us that forgets. In Compassionate Recovery, we try to be kind to all the parts of ourselves.

Create thoughts like the following or use these. Write them down in your journal.

I am kind to the part that forgot.

I feel compassion for the part of me that doesn't want to meditate.

I'm sending love to the part of me that feels anxiety when I sit still.

These are the kinds of thoughts we can generate in our self-empowering, self-compassion narrative as we try to learn to do the impossible task of training our traumatized minds not to run wild.

Notes

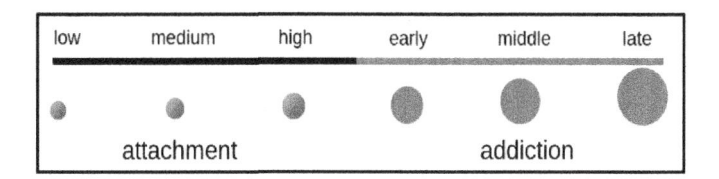

| low | medium | high | early | middle | late |

attachment　　　　　　　　addiction

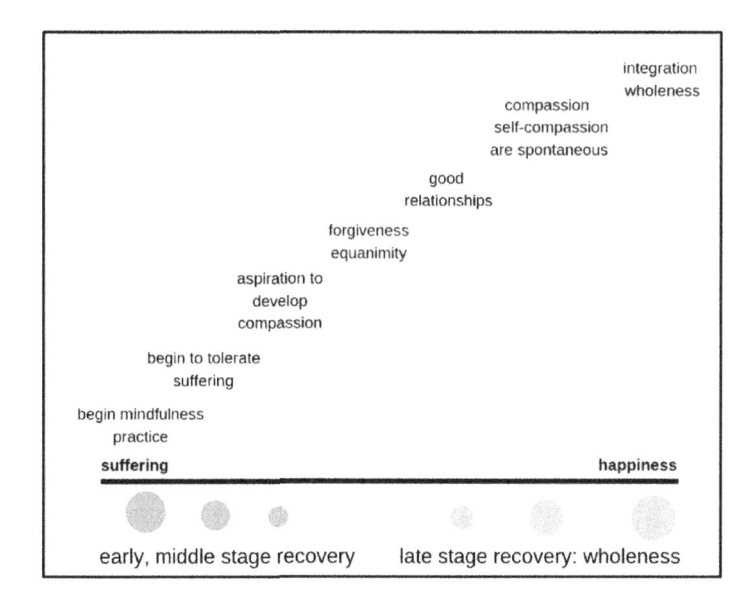

---

integration
wholeness

compassion
self-compassion
are spontaneous

good
relationships

forgiveness
equanimity

aspiration to
develop
compassion

begin to tolerate
suffering

begin mindfulness
practice

suffering　　　　　　　　　　　　　　　**happiness**

early, middle stage recovery　　late stage recovery: wholeness

Compassionate Recovery

Chapter 18
The Recovery-Mastery Spectrum

*"The day a man's mind shuts is
the day of his mental death."*
-Sir Arthur Conan Doyle[111]

Addiction is a disease, but we know that we don't have to see ourselves as diseased. Our disease of addiction is progressive, meaning that on the brain level, it gets worse over time, as we've discovered. Because our disease is progressive, our recovery must be progressive. It can't stop at the notion that we're sick addicts that will always be sick and that the best we can hope for is another day clean. If we get other stuff in life, that's the gravy. In Compassionate Recovery, we want to make our gravy with the tasty ingredients that give us meaning, purpose and connection.

We've covered a lot of material. The aim has been to give you an understanding which will fuel your drive to get out of suffering and into happiness. If

---

[111] 1930. Sir Arthur Conan Doyle created Sherlock Holmes. He was also an avid spiritualist. See The History of Spiritualism Vol 1, 2.

you've read to this point, congratulations. You've worked hard to understand your condition. The more knowledge we get, the more tools we have at our disposal. That means more chances, more hope, and a long-term scope. We can look ahead with a long-term view. A broken sense of self does not limit us. We are not broken. We are lights.

There's no need to hide in the shadows. It's time for us to shine. The good news is that your light is already on. The Light of Compassion will grow brighter within you and radiate to others as you do this work.

This chapter will take another look at the spectrums of attachment-addiction to recovery-mastery as one spectrum. We'll discuss healthy psychological attachment and attachment style. This has great implications for your relationship with the world, especially with a partner.

Once we see the process from attachment to addiction, we will shift the view to that of full-on individual human development. We'll end this edition with ideas for the future of a compassion-based community, in and out of recovery. This is all about how to put into practice what we've worked so hard to understand.

Attachment in Style

At the beginning of the attachment spectrum of attachment-addiction lies the issue of secure psychological attachment[112]. As an infant, we need a secure attachment to our primary caregiver. That happens in infancy, under normal conditions.

First, we need the right kind of caregiver. They stay close. They're attuned to us, which later teaches us to attune to ourselves. They respond to our deepest felt, non-verbal internal universe. We need them, feel for them, and are there, warm and responsive. This happens consistently, and we learn that we can explore the world around us without worrying about how close our caregiver is. When that doesn't happen, we learn separation anxiety instead, and our little nervous systems get jacked up from the get-go.

If normal attachment happens, we don't get anxious about getting too far away from mommy. We learn the world through safe, exploratory play with plenty of support. If we're experiencing ACEs, secure attachment is unlikely to be learned. We internalize a basic inner roadmap of what happens when we interact with others in a normal setting. Consistent stability should be the roadmap if we're expected to have healthy relationships with people in life. For addicts with ACEs, here's what you need to know. When we have a secure attachment, we develop an internal healthy relationship guidance

---

112 Bowlby (1979), cited in Weegmann, Martin & Cohen, R.. (2008). The Psychodynamics of Addiction. 10.1002/9780470713655.

system to recreate the same kind of secure relationships with others.

Our inner attachment roadmap is based on our experiences, especially in infancy. Remember, the earlier ACEs happen, the more serious the impact on development. Whatever our attachment imprint was early on is what our nervous systems will seek out for regulation—even if it is bad for us. The literature on this topic shows that the quality of relationships between a one-year-old and their caregiver consistently and accurately predicts later attachment style and other interpersonal characteristics. We all more or less marry our mothers at some point in our lives.

One of the critical issues for us is dealing with separation, grief, and loss. A whole volume could be written on this issue pertaining to addicts. For most of us, change is rough, even though it happens every day. Loss is devastating. We often spiral downward into addictions due to the overwhelming pain of grief. It takes us a long time to heal if we do at all. That can change right now. It doesn't have to be that way anymore if we do the work.

When we have a healthy inner roadmap for how to relate, forming new, healthy attachments is natural. But when we have the results of neglect and abuse, that's what feels like home. It's not home. We can make a new one with healthy attachments if we understand what this work is about, forming new brain circuits of empathy and compassion for others based on developing mindfulness and self-compassion for ourselves.

Our breath becomes the secure base as we meditate. The knowledge that we all share the same common humanity becomes the glint of recognition in our eyes that others see as if we know them. And we honestly want to get to know them, how they feel, what they've experienced, and what they dream. Our neural pathways of unhealthy attachments can't be erased, but we can burn in new ones starting today when it comes to healthy attachments.

When a secure attachment is thwarted, and we later develop addictions, we keep suckling at momma's booby with our drinks, pills, fixes, and drugs. She kicks us to the ground, and we scurry back, as desperate for love as an infant who's just been kicked can feel. Yet, as with all our addictions, the engagement in the object of our addiction will bring soothing relief, if not a good buzz.

The notion of attachment theory is that we develop attachment styles that shape our relations with other humans unless we get proactive and get some reshaping. We mammals need to form healthy attachments to our primary caregivers to survive and thrive. If we didn't get them in childhood, we could create them right now.

From our earlier perspective, problematic attachment is defined as an unhealthy bond, fixation, obsession, or preoccupation that causes life disruption. In Compassionate Recovery, addiction is defined as a form of severe attachment, but it's a form of insecure or anxious attachment from a clinical perspective. At the beginning of the spectrum is healthy attachment. When that doesn't happen, anxious or avoidant attachment styles form, with modulation between all three at different stages of life and the life of relationships. On the spectrum, *addiction is attachment gone wild.* Our unhealthy, anxious attachments can be to anything, a process, event, substance, or person.

Some theorists feel that addiction is a form of insecure or anxious attachment. In one study, addicts formed a trauma bond with their addiction, in this case heroin. The function of the heroin was thought to replace the bond that didn't form the way it should have with primary caregivers. In other words, if we attached well and in healthy ways with people who were there for us when we were young, and we *knew* they were there for us, we're less likely to form unhealthy attachments later on in life. But in the case of trauma, which means secure attachment was *not* the predominant experience, the chances are much higher that we'd form addictions of some kind.

A person isn't one attachment style all of the time. We have our phases. If our style is secure attachment, we're generally not the type to constantly look for validation. We see the world as friendly, not hostile. We work with people, not against them.

Avoidant attachment often develops from early childhood experiences of being overly dominated, abused, or smothered. It's characterized by being unable to let one's guard down, an inability to truly empathize with others, and problems with intimacy. Avoidant people tend to do just that, avoid feelings and closeness. We all do it at times, but this is the dominant style for some of us.

The other kind of attachment is anxious. Those with this style can be clingy, worried, codependent, and unable to be alone or comfortable in our own skin.

With practice, as we consider our attachment style, we can become more secure, more intimate, and more comfortable with ourselves and our relationships. All our practices here will help smooth out our attachments wherever they are on the spectrum.

Integration Practice: Relationship Inventory

Start a journal and a reading list about this topic. List and write in detail about the most important relationships at critical stages of your life: infancy, early childhood, adolescence, early adulthood, middle age, and senior. Your job is to discover the themes and patterns of your life in relation to others. What attachment styles reveal themselves between others in your family? In your life? How about between you and parts of yourself? What parts of you do you avoid or cling to? What parts are you secure with?

Don't try to do this in one day. It's a lifetime practice. Best to start now.

Notes

Chapter 19
Mastery

*"The person engaged in mastery of stress
may be likened to a sailor in a storm.
Stress is the storm, certainty is the compass,
change is the rudder, acceptance is the angle of the
sail set against the wind, and growth is the progress
toward a destination.
Mastery suggests that the sailor may not only avoid
being blown off course but may in fact use the wind
with such effectiveness as to make greater progress than
was expected."*
-Janet B. Younger, PhD, RN[113]

Before we get started, let's clarify that mastery in no way implies that you will control and enjoy your fentanyl addiction one day. If we haven't surrendered to the realities of our addictions, no mastery is possible. We're more likely to let our addiction run us into the grave than achieve anything. The result of addiction is the

---

[113] Younger JB. A theory of mastery. ANS Adv Nurs Sci. 1991 Sep;14(1):76-89. doi: 10.1097/00012272-199109000-00009. PMID: 1929239.

opposite of any kind of personal or spiritual mastery.

We haven't fully lost ourselves or wouldn't be here, now, on this road. But we haven't fully discovered ourselves yet, and that is why we move forward, each day, each moment in our recovery, and on our journey to mastery.

Mastery is conventionally defined as great skill, dominion, superiority, or knowledge. A master has command and control of their inner and outer scenarios. One aspect of mastery on our continuum of recovery is the way we handle, with all of our compassion and humanity, our response to a lifetime of ACEs and addictions. It's about the ways we develop competency, command, and control over the experience of toxic stress in our lives and the dysregulation it has caused.

The components of mastery include the miracle of how we come out better after weathering a lifetime of extensive suffering. What doesn't kill us makes us stronger, but it gives us a completely different view of ourselves and what life is and can be. We gain a sense of meaning that wouldn't be possible otherwise. It can lead to a life of fulfillment, happiness and yes, mastery of cool shit like tennis and how to make money on Instagram. But it's an inside job. It has been from the very start.

As we do this work, stay clean off our addictions and face the consciousness of our reality, we will no doubt experience backdraft. But instead of reacting against the monsters, we craft our new self-regulation plan that includes mindful self-compassion practice and high-intensity cardio training. That change in view and response to stress is a building block of mastery. The better we cope, the better we cope.

There is a place of suffering between a trauma experience, the fading of initial shock wears off and the sense of loss that sinks in, and a place of acceptance. We have many such places within us that await the ultimate relief of acceptance.

To cope means working through, confronting the feelings and back away, being in denial, and seeing through them. We get numb, and we get raw. But ultimately, the bad dreams subside; we stop compulsively reliving and repeating them consciously and unconsciously as we rebuild our relationship with our life and community.

Coping in and of itself, however, is not mastery. It's a component. Coping is about the work we do to deal with toxic stress. Mastery is the fruit of that effort that can be applied in ways that add confidence. Let us redefine our self-narrative into self-compassion and remap our worldview into one that sees and feels and acts on the common humanity everywhere.

As we develop mastery, we reconcile the relationship between our past reality and our current experience. As addicts with high ACEs, hair-trigger emotions and propensity to brace for impact rather than reach for the fruit, low hanging or otherwise, our amygdala constantly fires alarms based on frontal lobe memories that tell us the present is the past. But it isn't. Mastery is knowing that, in the moment, as it happens and changing the course of our emotional experience and those around us.

Mastery understands time and makes a new reality instead of being trapped in the old one. Mastery takes mindfulness, compassion, and other qualities. Mastery isn't an ego trip; it's not about dominating anyone, even our past. It's about being at peace and having enough certainty about the past that the forward path is evident as an Alabama[114] moon in August.

Mastery is about adjustment and alignment of our four dimensions. This helps us regulate and reduce anxiety. The more mastery we master, the more mastery we master. Mastery is dose-related. When we gain mastery of even one aspect that we're working on—this is a lifetime of work, not a weekend workshop—we reduce the anxiety firing non-stop from that trauma. One neurotransmitter at a time, amen.

In mastery, we learn to adapt to reality, not insist the world conform to ours. When we find mastery in some part of our journey, the goal is to emerge from

---

114 Or wherever moons are sold.

the suffering *"not demoralized and vulnerable, but healthy and stronger.[115]"*

The wisdom of the Greeks tells us that we gain peace through self-mastery and learning to accept what we cannot change and, most importantly, tolerate that loss. Most of us are likely to have some unprocessed loss of this nature that we can and will work on when the time is right on our road to mastery. However, we craft it, and however it turns out. Our recovery, our way.

I'm not saying we need to wake up at 0 Dark-thirty and run 10 miles on the treadmill. At the same time, we catch up with Elon Musk's latest tweets on our space watch and challenge Putin to a boxing match kind of mastery, though there is no apparent reason to put limits on it that would preclude such levels from being on the table.

It's more like my little emotional guts got chewed up and left wide open when I was an infant, and it went downhill from there. I had serious empathy issues that I couldn't turn off and stayed in allostatic overload way outside my window of tolerance most of the time. But I've worked on mastery in that area, one day at a time. It's getting better, slowly, slowly.

Each bit of ourselves that we heal as we go becomes part of our new neural network of compassionate healing. Instead of shrinking or fighting our inner and outer wars, we learn to live

---

[115] See epigraph to this chapter.

with our whole being. Something comes at us or feels like it, and we drop into flow mode, scoop, roll, sweep and duck, and boom, the knot of confusion and distress loosens and dissolves before it causes a migraine and a fight with your neighbor over the dog barking. Dogs are always right. Key takeaway: be nice to every dog every time, thanks.

Our roadmap is dynamic and in flux. We can study, learn, gain knowledge, and put it to use for ourselves and others. There is no reason to feel disconnected when we apply this. No matter how strange life can seem, we can cope with it. We're OK within ourselves. Chill af.

Does mastery mean that we don't have stress, make mistakes, cause suffering and forget the soy milk even after putting it on our list? Don't be ridiculous. You know better. Anyone who sells you that kind of guarantee is a scammer. We learn, we grow, and we do better. We spiral up. Life is suffering, and we can make it meaningful by making a difference, with compassion, in reducing the suffering in our world. Start now.

Mastery is creating ourselves on purpose. What happens when everything is suddenly snatched away? What do we have left? Masters have said that our only freedom is in our attitude and the decisions that we make. Decide on generosity. Commit to patience. See things through with diligence and focus. Do it all in the space of compassionate mindfulness. Watch for opportunities to make people feel way better than before you came along. Make that moment. Make that meaning. This is how we connect in Compassionate Recovery. It's the opposite of alienation, disconnection, and shame. And way more fun. Did I mention that there are some instructions for having a Compassion Circle at the end? Talk about fun!

The more mastery we gain over our emotional regulation and general stress management, the safer we feel. The safer we feel, the more resources and compassion we can effortlessly switch on because we've practiced.

Mastery means we're not ruled by our demons anymore. We talked. Everybody came to dinner, and we all listened to each other's viewpoints and decided they were all valid. There is room for everyone. We celebrated with herbal tea and fart jokes. Mastery over some of our challenging aspects is hard work.

The good news is that when we develop mastery in some areas, our brains learn new capabilities to interact and cope with the world that we live in. The result is feeling less threatened and more capable of finding satisfaction. Yes, you can.

Being satisfied with this moment, rather than the moment that should have been, is mastery. When we know who we are, we no longer must reach for the light when we hear a cat howl. Cats are great too; feed one.

When we discover our vulnerability and humanity, we no longer need to hold up the fantasy that we must be somehow invulnerable human beings. It's not possible. What is possible is that through our compassionate self-healing practice, we gain mastery of our heart space which results in a decrease in self-loathing, thereby triggering some oxytocin without ever having to leave the comfort of your own home.

No longer trapped in hyperarousal, ready to kill or be killed in any grocery store altercation over toilet paper, we learn to dwell in the space of mastery, to direct our energies to higher aspirations toward our expanding potential as living, compassionate Beings of Light.

Mastery is making it this far. No matter how much you've been through, here you are. Me too. That's what's up. We don't have to do it alone.

When we gain regulation through mindfulness tempered with wisdom and compassion, we don't react compulsively when our triggers pop up out of nowhere.

In mastery, we don't long for what is lost. Instead, we have the confidence to form psychologically healthy, compassionate attachments rather than take emotional hostages. The energy we put toward holding on to toxic relationships with ourselves and others is freed up to make new, healthy connections based on listening and caring rather than tricking and stealing like an emotional black crow.

Mastery reflects the old with the new and is grateful for the ability to create who we want to be. Do you. It's the new you.

Practice:
Stance of Power

Stand with your feet separated. Bend your knees a little. Push down into your feet, so you feel rooted. Lift your torso from the waist up. If you're unable to stand, modify whatever way you can to feel strong.

This is your power stance. You are not a victim. You have power, the power of compassion. Say the following words.

I am self-empowered.

I live in the heart of compassion.

My choices are mine to make.

I allow myself the freedom and self-compassion to choose *not* to practice my attachments, just for today.

Breathe in deeply. Feel a warm, rosy-colored light at your heart center. Exhale, let go of wounds. Let go of suffering. Repeat a few times, slowly. Say the words silently to yourself.

I am self-empowered.

I live in compassion.

I am at peace.

I am strong.

From this center, I live and move and have my being.

May all beings be free of suffering.
May we all know our own strength.
May all of us live from a Wise Mind.

Write your own version as time goes on. Start with just one thing and build from there. Build what you need most to hear into your script. Make it a self-compassion, self-empowerment activity with others. Actively change your brain and your emotional state and the way others interact with you.

Components of Mastery

Everything is easier to understand when we break things down into parts. These are based on research-based patterns in the literature of people recovering from trauma which reveals elements as key components of the process of mastery that we are involved in.

Certainty

A necessary component of mastery that enables us to plan, make decisions, and move forward on our roadmap, certainty means that you adopt a view that you can live with, then live with it. There's no need for doubt because you've worked it out in advance. The view may be something like that we all share a common humanity. Based on that view, actions follow. The view with this kind of masterful certainty isn't foolish. It's based on the evidence of all our life philosophy, trial and error experimentation, and contemplation of the universe to compare and reflect the old, less compassionate internal representation of you with the new, super warm, and approachable outward manifestation of you.

That point of mastery happens when the confidence of certainty arrives. This certainty provides you with the clarity, confidence, and vision to articulate your mission in life. The task is kindness. Start with you. Mastery is knowing that we deserve self-compassion.

Change

When we have the courage to change, we notice that what we can deal with changing right now is right there in front of us. Real change requires real compassion and real effort. If nothing changes, nothing changes. One micro-adjustment today can put you in a whole new place five years from now. Life is problematic. Masters are problem solvers. Achieving change means dealing with environmental stressors by cushioning their blow to our dopamine reuptake system with consistent training in mindful self-care. We make changes happen that are in favor of our well-being.

When we go through tremendous challenges and survive to make positive changes, the transformation brings new skills that weren't part of the old-school toolkit. We craft some new-school tools.

Mastery is knowing or making, the right tool for the

job. We learn to welcome and even initiate changes in our lives.

Change is an inside job, and our insides match our outsides when we make authentic change that is true to our heart of empathy and compassion.

Acceptance

We've lost a lot. When we come to a place where the grieving process is complete, the voice of mastery sounds like:

I acknowledge the truth of the events in my life
And admit what cannot be changed
My heart is open to experience the impact of that realization
I give up hopeless causes and expectations
I've let go and am free of longing for what has been lost,
For I have grieved all my losses
All the changes that are required, are of myself
I have new goals, new relationships and new sources of comfort and ease.
I am free of fear and despair.
Mastery is acceptance of the way it is, while knowing what can and can't be changed. For example, we cannot change events that have already occurred at a previous moment.

Growth

The best defense is not a good offense. Not in this game. When we refine mastery, we learn new competencies and become stronger with a greater sense of purpose than before we did the work. Life got much less confusing. The most drama we get into is on Law and Order. When we're in mastery, we grow. The past doesn't keep us locked to a pole like an abused and neglected dog. If you see a dog that's suffering, take compassionate action. When we're not locked by the past's traumatic feelings or numbness, our energy is free to move forward with our whole, mindful being.

This free energy moves us into our next-level aspiration since we're not on defense lock-down mode down in the emotional bunker under a seemingly innocuous potato farm anymore, Dorothy.

The way we go after and manage growth is mandatory for mastery. As new situations and stresses appear before us on our road of recovery, we become clearer. Even in situations that threaten us, we're regulated enough to protect ourselves. Life is no longer a threat to our survival. Now, that's growth!

The result is that we're equipped for a compassion mission. Our experience can be used to offer compassionate service to ease and end suffering for other beings in this world, especially for those who've walked a similar path.

These four components can't be separated, but they can be understood relative to the process of mastery of one's own internal response to stress in the past, present, and future and knowing which is which. We must have some certainty to change and find acceptance. Without both, we couldn't grow.

Mastery is already available within yourself. It is attainable and expandable to anything that you want it to be. You're already doing it. That's what you need to know about mastery.

Integration Practice: Self-compassion Certainties

Make a list in your journal of the certainty of your value. Here are some examples. As always, create your own.

I am of value.

I deserve to exist.

My view of my situation is congruent with that of my circle of safety.

The way I view my life to date is not distorted.

My insides match what's going on around me.

I'm committed to my decision to grow.

My legs are in a power stance.

My tone of voice declares how things are with assuredness.

If I'm certain of nothing else, it's that I don't want to go back to the way it was before recovery.

Extra credit: What are some of the ways you've attempted to change events that can't be changed? How have you stood in the way of your own growth? What are you not willing to accept? Be detailed.

Write about it. Share about it. Meet with some recovery friends to sit mindfully with it.

Notes

Chapter 20
Practicing the Principles

"There is no difficulty that enough love will not conquer;
No disease that enough love will not heal;
No door that enough love will not open;
No gulf that enough love will not bridge;
No wall that enough love will not throw down;
No sin that enough love will not redeem. . .
It makes no difference how deeply seated may be the trouble,
How hopeless the outlook, how muddled the tangle, how great the mistake—a sufficient realization of love will dissolve it all. . . if only you could love enough, you would be the happiest and most powerful being in the world."
-Emmet Fox

PRIN'CIPLE, n. L. principium, beginning.
1. In a general sense, the cause, source, or origin of anything; that from which a thing proceeds; as the principle of motion; the principles of action.

The principle is the essential element of something. It is the ground and foundation from which any worthy and substantive declaration about life must be made. Principle is active. Like the Law of Gravity, a principal can be tested. It works if you work it.

When principles are found to be repeatable and reliable, they become general truths or laws, such as the principle of non-harming or *ahimsa*[116]. Principles are set on a serious of conclusions such as harming others causes suffering. I don't want to suffer, and neither do the other beings.

Principles become the answer to questions such as, "What should I do?" and "Is there a good way to handle that?".

We've discussed most of the tools we'd want to use in a recovery mission based on compassion. We can return to the explanations and study repeatedly until the things we need to understand become clear enough to put into practice. As we go, the principles are ready to be put into use right now. No days of sobriety are required. No special hat or tattoo. Best of all, no experiences are necessary. You've already lived all the experiences you'll ever need to make Compassionate Recovery work for you.

Elements of Compassion

Dr. Margaret Cullen of Stanford's Compassion Institute breaks down compassion into four

---

[116] Sanskrit, principle of yoga

elements. None of these elements of compassion need to come first or last. They're all interwoven and can be approached in any order. The ideas align with what we've been working on with our physical, mental, emotional, and spiritual selves.

Cognitive Element

This is a mental process. Compassion has a cognitive aspect that is engaged when we practice mindful awareness. In this regard, we acknowledge and ultimately accept that suffering happens for ourselves and others. This creates a shift in perspective as we notice that suffering is present. Because everything is entwined, the mental is also infused with and affected by the other elements. The cognitive aspect is essential to consider because it's with our thinking mind that we can make a conscious choice to think or act compassionately. We can envision or feel all the brain circuitries involved in these processes. If we can coach ourselves out of troubled emotional waters through conscious intention and directed thought towards something like compassion, it will guide us. Without the cognitive element of compassion, we wouldn't be able to think through the helping strategies and problem-solving that we need to help others.

Emotional Element

When we practice compassion, we improve our capacity to develop empathy on an emotional level. As we learned earlier, empathy is the capacity to feel for others as if their pain is our own. This is the dynamic quality of feeling compassion, so it should be dealt with in a non-attached way. Addicts can easily be addicted to emotional states, such as distress, longing, resentment, and depression. An addict who is an empath can have trouble dealing with the experience they have in their bodies because they pull in so much energy from other people. It's important to be aware of these tendencies to develop a healthy approach to having empathy and compassion without getting fatigued or distressed.

Motivational Element

When we set an intention like the wish for others to be relieved of suffering, this is the motivational aspect of compassion. We use our intention to fuel compassion, and in turn, our compassionate experience nourishes our motivation to continue wishing for or working for others to be free of suffering. In Buddhism and other systems, meditation on suffering, the impermanence of all phenomena, and even our own impending death helps to create the motivation to be a compassionate person.

To the extent that we can continue to deceive ourselves into thinking that everything's fine, we will remain mired in the bottomless swamp of suffering. If we're busy distracting ourselves from our pain by self-medicating with drugs and alcohol or our other addictions, we prolong the inevitable suffering that comes not only with addiction, but with life itself. When we consciously choose to encounter the suffering that is the underlying reality of our lives, the process of compassion can begin.

Behavioral Element

With the behavioral element of our compassion, we learn to practice responsiveness, or a readiness to act to alleviate suffering. We walk what we talk. That's right; we walk it like we talk it. As the adage goes, we're judged by our behavior, not our intentions. Action is key. Are we going to act in a compassionate manner all the time? Nope. But we can stay mindful and use our cognitive, emotional, and motivational elements of compassion to drive our actions.

Our motivations, feelings, and actions come from a place of service and healing rather than grabbing what we can get.

Though we've already "defined" Compassion, it will be helpful to keep our minds open in a spirit of active inquiry. If we think we already know something, we can close ourselves off from learning more deeply. There's an old saying in sales, "Stay green and grow. Ripen and rot." The less we *know* about something, the more open we can be to learning.

In my experience, the study and practice of compassion as a principle have no end. I've been at it for decades, and I can say that I'm constantly surprised, both at my capacity not to get it and my ability to somehow, often suddenly, feel it on clearly and deeply.

As we practice compassion this way, we increase understanding with our whole being and an open mind of inquiry. By default, resistance gives way to an increase in compassion. When we increase our capacity for compassion, we deepen our connections to ourselves and the world.

Addicts, no matter how social, are generally at the core, very disconnected and alienated. The more we learn to connect compassionately with others on a genuine, authentic level, the better we get at healing. This is the theme of Compassionate Recovery.

The Principles of Compassionate Recovery

The Generosity of Compassion

May I release attachments by making offerings to others in need.

May I relinquish self-centered thoughts and focus on how I can help a living being who needs compassion.

May I practice enough mindfulness to be fully present for myself and others.

May I be generous with my whole being—with all beings.

The Patience of Compassion

May I be patient with myself because this work is hard.

May I have the patience to pause until the anger passes, however long it takes.

May I be patient with the process of growth and healing through spirals up and down.

Even if I falter in patience for myself, may I always find it for others.

Compassion with Diligence

There is no inertia in compassion, for it flows freely from my heart.

May I never abandon this.

However many steps it takes, I vow to complete my path.

May I always remember this.

May the energy to practice compassion be inexhaustible, as compassion is inexhaustible.

The path takes commitment and hard work.

May I never give up, no matter what.

Compassionate Focus

May I focus with my whole being on the path of recovery.

May the actions of my body be focused on service to end suffering.

May the intentions of my mind be focused on bringing happiness to others.

May the focus always be on compassion, as unwavering as the focus on addiction.

The Ethics of Compassion

May all my words bring comfort and ease to everyone that meets me.

May I be as diligent in my ethics when alone as in front of others.

The light in my heart knows what will cause suffering or ease it. May I keep the flame lit.

May all my actions bring peace and safety to all beings that I encounter.

The Wisdom of Compassion

May the actions of my body be compassionate to myself and others.

May I cultivate warm and compassionate feelings toward myself and others.

When my compassion grows weary from giving, may I practice self-compassion and take care of myself

In the core of my heart-mind, may I always remember our common humanity.

Notes

Chapter 21
Compassionate Communication

"Every criticism, judgment, diagnosis, and expression of anger is the tragic expression of an unmet need. What I want in my life is compassion, a flow between myself and others based on a mutual giving from the heart."
-Marshall B. Rosenberg[117]

Compassionate communication is the basis for supportive, non-stressful, and un-toxic relationships. In recovery, relationships are also key to our survival. We need to be better at them. Compassionate communication skills are the most important tool that we can have in our road kit.

This chapter is meant to introduce you to this well-studied topic with an extraordinary amount of literature and training. What follows is a down and dirty synopsis based on notes from in-person workshops, training videos, and readings by

---
[117] Nonviolent Communication: A Language of Life, Marshall B. Rosenberg, PhD

Marshall Rosenberg, Ph.D.. He spent his life developing Non-Violent Communication as a way to communicate compassionately.

You're encouraged to look into this further because it's worth learning it to the point where it's spontaneous. Some social media groups will help you connect with another person learning compassionate communication. Spending time with a trained, compassionate communicator firmly grounded in it as a life practice is the best way to learn this.

In my experience, even awkwardly and sparingly applied, these tools have changed the course of interactions with human beings in ways that I would have never thought possible. The principles are in perfect alignment with Compassionate Recovery.

The process involves four areas to practice; observations, feelings, needs, and requests[118]. First, we say what we observe with our five senses, which we find disturbing to our wellbeing. "When I see you are speaking with someone else when I'm waiting for you," is an observation, whereas "Hey, asshole, do you not know who you're dealing with?" conveys judgment and is otherwise uncompassionate in its approach. Many skills can be practiced and developed in all these areas. Good communication means avoiding stress that can trigger us into the funnel or other dark places.

---

[118] Note: whining and cajoling are not on the list

The key elements to remember are that observations are distinctly different from interpretations, analyses, judging, criticizing, and labeling. The key is to make neutral statements that are based on objective facts. I see this; I heard that. Make it factual.

Moral judgments are not observations. When we evaluate someone else, it's an example of our own unmet needs. Instead of causing defensiveness and resistance with someone we're trying to get to show up on time or making them comply out of guilt, we start with observation, not blame.

The next part of compassionate communication is to express our feelings in a non-aggressive way. Through the practices that we've covered in this book, we can develop the ability to use our brain's discernment circuits to discern how we feel. Then we choose an accurate, fact-based way of stating that feelings related to our unmet needs. The base reaction for most hair-trigger sensitive addicts would be to express our anger as, "It really pisses me off when you make me wait." The honest way to take responsibility for our feelings would be, "I feel anger in my chest when this happens."

Remember not to take the victim role when expressing your feelings. Recovery is about taking responsibility, starting with owning our own feelings. We're still in low-key attack dog mode if we use action words like disrespected, underappreciated, or ignored.

When we start with an observation instead of an accusation, the person on the receiving end has less reason to put up their deflector shields. As we share our feelings without blaming them on the other person, they can empathize with us. Then we can talk about what's going on and our needs are not being met.

We need to know what our needs are to know when they're not being satisfied. It's not about what we think we deserve. It's about what we need. Needs can be things that we value, like timeliness. If we say, "Because I value timeliness," it expresses our need for it to be respected as one of your base values. "It would make my life better if you can help me out on the time thing, bro."

The key is to know the difference between our blame games and manipulation strategies and the universal, life-sustaining values that motivate us to be on time. Be mindful not to attach your value to the other person. You don't need Bob's timeliness. You need timeliness. It's always about our unmet needs, not Bob.

Since the communication is stable, we're now in a position to get down to requesting what we need for our wellbeing. Remember, the anger isn't about the other person being late. It's about our value of timeliness is an unmet need in this case. "For my wellbeing, would you be willing to commit to being on time when we meet?"

That's the fourth skill, asking for a concrete action that will get your needs met and doesn't get the other person riled up. A request differs from a demand in that we don't use shame, guilt, or bribes. We make a present moment request that is clear and specific. "If we agree on 7 pm, would you be willing to commit to that?"

We can ask if they've heard you or what they heard. Ask how they feel about what you're communicating. Listen to the answers. Remember, the difference between an honest request and a manipulative demand is that you can take the word "no," as a possible answer. If you have expectations, those are implicit demands. The work of recovery is about letting go of attachments, so when making your request, let go of the results. The exception would be in the event of an emergency.

Practice:
What do I observe?

What do I observe; see, hear, remember, and imagine that is free from my evaluations and does or does not contribute to my well-being?

Practice:
What do I feel?

When your needs are satisfied:

Affectionate, compassionate, friendly, loving, Open-hearted, sympathetic, tender, warm

Confident, empowered, open, proud, safe, secure

Engaged, absorbed, alert, curious, engrossed, enchanted, entranced, fascinated, interested, intrigued, involved, spellbound, stimulated

Inspired, amazed, awed, wonder, excited, animated, aroused, astonished, eager, energetic, enthusiastic, giddy, invigorated, lively, passionate, surprised, vibrant

Exhilarated, blissful, ecstatic, elated, enthralled, exuberant, radiant, thrilled

Grateful, appreciative, moved, thankful, touched

Hopeful, expectant, encouraged, optimistic

Joyful, amused, delighted, glad, happy, jubilant, pleased

Peaceful, calm, clear-headed, comfortable, centered, content, fulfilled, mellow, quiet, relaxed, relieved, satisfied, serene, still, tranquil

When your needs are not satisfied:

Afraid, apprehensive, dread, foreboding, frightened, mistrustful, panicked petrified, scared, suspicious, terrified, wary, worried

Annoyed, aggravated, dismayed, disgruntled, displeased, exasperated, frustrated, impatient, irritated, irked

Angry, enraged, furious, incensed, indignant, irate, livid, outraged, resentful

Aversion, animosity, appalled, contempt, disgusted, dislike, hate, horrified, hostile, repulsed

Confused, ambivalent, baffled, bewildered, dazed, hesitant, lost, mystified, perplexed, puzzled, torn

Disconnected, alienated, aloof, apathetic, bored, cold, detached, distant, distracted, indifferent, numb, removed, uninterested, withdrawn

Fatigue, beat, burnt out, depleted, exhausted, lethargic, listless, sleepy, tired, weary, worn out

Sad, depressed, dejected, despair, despondent, disappointed, discouraged, gloomy

Tense, anxious, cranky, distressed, edgy, irritable, jittery, nervous, overwhelmed, restless, stressed out

Practice:
What do I need?

Connection: acceptance, affection, appreciation, belonging, cooperation, communication, closeness, community, companionship, compassion, consideration, consistency, empathy, inclusion, intimacy, love, mutuality, nurturing, respect/self-respect, safety, security, stability, support, to know and be known, to see and be seen to understand and be understood trust, warmth

Honesty; authenticity, integrity, presence

Play, joy, and humor

Peace; beauty, communion, ease, equality, harmony, inspiration, order

Physical Wellbeing: air, food, water, exercise, rest, sexual, safety, shelter, touch

Meaning; awareness, a celebration of life, challenge, clarity, competence, consciousness, contribution, creativity, discovery, efficacy, effectiveness, growth, hope, learning, mourning, participation, purpose, self-expression, stimulation, understanding

Autonomy, choice, freedom, independence, space, spontaneity

Practice:
Write Your Request

You need to know three main points when making your needs-based, demand-free request. First, make sure that your request is clear, positive, and concrete, precise action that you're asking for. Second, the request should be something that can be done right there, right then. If the person says no, chill out.

Frame your words in the positive rather than the negative. Instead of, "don't do that," try "if you did this, it would be helpful for me." Try it out in a safe, test case scenario. It works. Here's a key point. When you get a "no," it's not a bad thing. See it as an opportunity to empathize. Ask questions. Listen.

Repeat back what they say and ask if you've heard them correctly. It will open doors.

These are the main ideas of how to communicate with compassion. It may save your life because addiction is life-threatening, and connections are life-sustaining. Work through the three topics in practice to prepare for your request. Try writing these out first, then practice them with a friend in recovery before attempting them in the real world. Write out your request.

You're doing great!

Notes

Chapter 22
Compassionate Community

Do not be daunted
by the insurmountability of the world's grief.
Do justly, now.
Love mercy, now.
Walk humbly, now.
You are not obligated to complete the work
but neither are you free to abandon it.
-The Talmud

Suffering has no limitations. But neither does compassion. In its true nature, absolute compassion has no limits whatsoever. The only limitations to compassion are those that we impose with our attachments to self and other obsessions. We can make our world as small as we want. But why die alone, drunk in a trailer when several billion people out there share the same common humanity? Every single person has a heart.

We all suffer, and we would all benefit from a smile and a hug. We can connect in unbelievable ways with amazing people when we train ourselves to be free of limitations in empathy and compassion.

Back in the day, we used to say that wherever two or more are gathered, we have a recovery community. Before Zoom, we sometimes held meetings with two guys and a pot of coffee when living in an isolated area.

In Compassionate Recovery, we expand the sense of community in ways as important as one addict talking to another, but we work on creating relationships that are just as strong by using the tools we've been talking about. When the individual heals, they go out and spread the love. But it's not just with our recovery peeps. What if we think of community as starting with one human being connecting authentically with all the various concentric social circles we live in, from the family to the community to wider society? What if that being is you?

The human tendency is to cling together in tribes for survival. Since the dawn of humankind, we've been brutally tearing each other apart because of us vs. them or in-group/out-group mentality. That needs to evolve right now. It's just us now. Here, together. We need each other.

This view of recovery goes into an expansion of human potential in recovery to personal mastery of whatever you can dream of and are willing to work for. As you work on your journey, you'll be in community with the other beings who live here. You can positively affect every single one of them because the change starts in you. Instead of shame, fear, and self-doubt, you put energy out from your home base of self-compassion, empathy for others, mindful emotional self-discernment, generosity, and the other base principles of this book.

Community is a process. It begins when two people make eye contact. The dynamics change. Community isn't about one person's view; it's about sharing what we share in common and learning about what is unique to us.

Community is a practice. The sense of sharing a common bond of suffering is key in recovery. But we can connect on so much more than that. Even though much of the work can be done alone, the benefit of social support cannot be overstated, as we know. Collaboration with the parts of ourselves helps us collaborate with others.

Community is seen as a practice principle. At any given point, we can pose the question, "Does this serve the community?" Through an increased sense of openness to compassion principles, Compassionate Recovery members can play a vital role in those in and out of recovery to connect and share a path of compassion. This is very different than the typical feeling of in-group, out-group that happens in every type of human organization. In the way we're viewing it here, everyone is our "real" family, not just those closest to us or with the same political or other values.

Compassionate Recovery is based on the integration of principles into our daily lives. It's about retraining ourselves. We learn how to create strong bonds with our closest recovery peers, but we also get right out there and start making a difference in the world.

We are inclusive in our approach. Addicts and ACEs survivors have been marginalized enough. Everyone is welcome. That means everyone. There is no need for gay meetings over here and heroin meetings down there, and meetings for lawyers only. There is no need. We are not broken. We don't live in shame. We are out of the shadows and in the community. Get used to it.

Compassionate Recovery is universal. It is intended to work with:

Religious groups
Recovery Meetings
Women's Shelters
LGBTQ Community Groups
Men's Support Groups
Treatment Centers
Yoga Teacher Training
Compassion Training
Your Book Club!

Compassionate Recovery believes that compassion is a universal tool that can be developed and applied across racial, religious, gender, and political boundaries. The practices are meant to work well with other approaches, not against them.

Please feel free to use this material in your existing group. There should be no problem. If there is, grab a couple of like-minded people and try some of the other community ideas here. We're trying to have some fun over here.

Compassionate Recovery can have different types of meetups, but it's not a 'meeting based' system. It's an integration system where you as the individual integrate with yourself and the world in different, fun and interesting ways. Here are a few ideas, but please create new ones for yourself and your community.

Compassionate Meet-outs

Excursions to interesting places.
Volunteering where it's needed most.
Journaling sessions.
Nature walks.
Camping trips.
Dance, drum, or singing circles.
Pottery Barn
Dog Parks
Yoga or fitness class
Wellness lunch
Spa

Mindful focus groups for specific topics such as a type of addiction or issue would also be helpful, if it doesn't detract from the inclusiveness of the whole community, as principle.

Mindful Meet-ins

Mindful meet-ins:
Silent meditation only
Meditation and sharing
Guest speaker
Mindful walking through; parks, streets, malls
Online sessions
Reading groups

Armed Services

Addiction and trauma-related disorders are a problem in the military. For decades, the effects of war were kept out of the research because PTSD makes war look bad. Veterans are often given powerful opioids to deal with injuries. The number of suicides among veterans with addiction and PTSD was so high that on May 21st, 2019, the United States House of Representatives unanimously voted to pass a bill[119] requiring the VA to study holistic treatment methods for mental health.

---

119 H.R. 2359 "The Whole Veteran Act will require VA to provide Congress with an analysis of the accessibility and health outcomes of each of the following services at VA medical facilities (including community-based outpatient clinics, vet centers, and community living centers): massage, chiropractic services, whole health clinician services and coaching, acupuncture, healing touch, whole health group services, guided imagery, equine services, mediation and

We can bring a non-religious, principles-based recovery program to the military and all who suffer from trauma. This book was written with the men and women who serve our country in mind. Together, we can collaborate and create a compassionate community where it is needed, inside and outside organizations and institutions.

Correctional Facilities

In the years since The 12-Step Buddhist was published, I've received more emails from people who read the book while doing time than any other group of people. I still get regular emails from people who tell me they've got some years sober and read the book in prison. I didn't know about that when I wrote that book. It's different now.

I've never done time, but I remember something that my first AA sponsor, "Prison Larry," used to say. He said he'd been freed from the prison of his own mind by getting sober and working the program. In the recovery that some friends have found in prisons, it's clear that the work is an inside job, whether we're inside or not.

If you're locked up, this book was written with you in mind. Please stay tuned for a way to connect with a free book and mentor program that we're developing.

---

yoga, among other holistic treatments." -https://lamb.house.gov/media/press-releases/house-passes-lambs-whole-veteran-act

Non-English-Speaking Communities

This book is open for translation into any language. If you need it in your country and have someone who will do the translation, contact us at feedback@compassionaterecovery.US so we can try to work it out. Spanish is first on the list at the moment.

Compassionate Recovery Community Concepts

- Based on compassion with the understanding of trauma as a strong correlate to addiction and its role in the recovery process
- To be of service to all beings is the attitude.
- Unlimited. Welcomes any valid tools
- Integrates principles and practices based on new science
- Begins with meditation as a foundation
- Begins with a premise of universality and openness that prevents underlying rigidity that can spawn fundamentalist thinking
- Works to dissolve ego attachment using up to date information as well as tried and true principles
- Inclusive. No identification of a particular addiction is required or encouraged. Anyone can participate if *they* feel they have an

attachment that is problematic at any place on the spectrum of attachment-addiction
- We are poly or non-theistic
- There is no hierarchy
- We use sensitive language that is neutral and welcoming to women, people of color, LGBTQ, and others who consider themselves marginalized
- There are no steps to work in order.
- There are principles that can be dipped into and practiced in any amount at any time
- We are open to
  - change
  - cooperation with trained facilitators and community leaders
  - any literature that provides insight and support conducive to compassion
  - all issues that address the total human and the ultimate evolution of people and the planet
- Our work is heart-centered over intellectually oriented
- Recovery is seen as a complex path for complex people. The tools used are simple, but the individual is never minimized, and problems are not over simplified
- We welcome those with secular and/or spiritual beliefs or none at all

- There are no gurus, but compassionate leaders are encouraged to train in the principles to guide others with humility

12 Steps of Compassionate Recovery

This book is not a steps-in-order deal. It's meant to be dipped into anywhere and anytime that you need it. Understand that it may make more sense to put in a step format for those of us who would like to connect the principles of Compassionate Recovery to a more familiar model. Consider these steps that follow as a loose guideline. You should rewrite these in a meaningful way for you, and that you connect with. As discussed, meaning and connection are recovery survival tools: your recovery, your way.

1. I have power over my actions and choices. Due to attachments and addictions, my life has become mf unmanageable.

2. In each fresh moment, I regularly renew what I have come to believe: that kindness, compassion, and love are the true powers of the universe.

3. I make consistent decisions to base all my actions on compassion.

4. In an ongoing inventory of actions and attitudes, I seek vigilance to record all events that come up where I could not regulate my emotions.

5. I stay honest with myself and others. I often discuss my thoughts, feelings, intentions, and actions with my Circle of Safety.

6. After reviewing all the suffering I have caused and endured, I finally got ready to drop the rock and join the mindful walking path.

7. I stay mindful and compassionate, enjoying the walk.

8. I listed all the harms and bad intentions that are the core of my fears. I often contemplate the actual magnitude of harm my intentions and actions have caused others.

9. I meditate and practice compassion for others. Where I've caused harm, I work on making it right with those beings, however, they want. I constantly work to watch my mind and my hands. I try sincerely to make things as right as possible and not repeat the same patterns.

10. I try to stay in self-compassion with regular practice. Each day, I study, reflect, share, and try to be free of ego.

11. I am a meditator. I take the practice seriously. I might even learn pranayama.

12. Together with my community, I stay committed to recovery and live my life based on principles of mindfulness, compassion, generosity, patience, diligence, and wisdom. Wherever any being is suffering, I empathize and try to help.

May I act swiftly to free all beings from suffering and its causes.

May all beings live freely in wisdom and happiness.

Compassionate Recovery Group Guidelines

Recommended

Listen actively.
Offer compassion as support.
Keep sharing the practice or principle at hand.
Be a peer.
Respect the rights of others to share.
Respect the time of others.
Be gut-level honest.
Take risks.
Trust!
Empathize!

If there's a topic, focus on it. Practice common humanity. We're all in this together. This is the entire point.

We don't go into detail about specific beliefs or war stories. We rehash the experiences of trauma that have affected us so deeply. We don't want to trigger others.

In a Compassionate Recovery get-together, we study principles and practices and share our experiences with the healing. This allows people of different backgrounds and orientations to come together in a compassionate, safe community. Everyone can feel safe when we look for the similarities, not the differences, but celebrate those differences!

Safety is a key component to our healing, so we ask that members work diligently to ensure a safe space for everyone. You are responsible

Not recommended

No fixing.

No advice giving.

Don't teach when you share. Share your own experience with the practice or principle for that meeting.

No therapizing.

No crosstalk.

No group hijacking.

No war stories or drug-alogues.

In Compassionate Recovery, we share our feelings around the practices and principles.

To not alienate anyone, your specific addiction is your business. We're all in this to heal. We focus on the commonalities and celebrate our differences.

Please maintain confidentiality.

No fragrances/aromatherapy nor smelly foods, please.

Please be respectful and accepting of diversity.

One person speaks at a time.

Please be supportive, but don't problem-solve for others.

Please, no recording allowed.

Be kind to yourself above all else! If your compassion doesn't include yourself, it's incomplete!

This is not therapy. We share based upon our direct experiences in the here and now. Nevertheless, if something does get triggered within you, we will support you.

Speak from your own experience.

Please keep a supportive intention for all in the group, including yourselves.

Actively listen. Your presence is a gift!

Mindfully share as to not monopolize.

Okay, to choose to remain silent.

No crosstalk.

Please silence your cell phones and beepers.

Visiting is encouraged outside the room before the meeting. At the time of arriving inside the space, let us aim to keep an "honoring attitude," meaning to honor one another's practice and our own, a time to unwind and settle in. So, when you cross the threshold into the room, please mindfully land softly into your chairs and keep in mind that others may be practicing. Feel free to socialize inside and out of the room during the breaks and after the meeting.

In addition to group activities, please commit to a daily home practice. If you miss a day, don't beat yourself up. Try again tomorrow!

What follows is a sample format for a meet-in. This is in no way carved in stone. Feel free to switch things around or include it in your regular recovery group. This is open to interpretation. There will be more in the follow-up workbook. Please check the website compassionterecovery.US as well for more content.

Compassionate Recovery Circle

Setting: Set up a circle with comfortable seating on cushions and chairs. You'll need a meditation bell, which can be from your smartphone. An electric candle or nice soft light arrangement, flowers, pictures of ancestors, sobriety coins, and things to let go of written on little paper can all go around the light. If you're outdoors and have a safe fire pit, that can also be used. No fires inside, ever. Please.

If everyone likes incense or essential oil diffuser scents, those can be used to enhance the setting. Set a timer for no more than one hour. Once seated, ring the bell, and begin with a full minute of stillness to set an intention for what you want to work on. Next, read the welcome, everyone.

Welcome.

If you struggle with anything from difficult attachments to full-blown addictions or attachments gone wild, you are welcome here. Our main principles are self-compassion, mindfulness, and compassion. We practice using our practice to help others. We train our hearts and minds to do this.

From there, we can bring true compassion to our community.

Read the Compassionate Recovery Concepts.

Go around the circle for a one-word check-in on a physical, mental, emotional, or spiritual plane—just one.

Add a reading of your choosing. Keep it short. No more than a few sentences so that everyone can absorb the meaning.

Sit for 20 minutes of stillness. Collective practices can be done as an option instead of stillness.

Optional sharing on what came up for you or what you're working on. Use three descriptive words or share for three minutes.

The designated leader for this session will share last.

Read the Compassionate Recovery Principles.

Dedicate the merits.

Caught in the self-centered dream, only suffering.

Holding to self-centered thoughts.

Each moment, life as it is, the only teacher.

Being just this moment, compassion's way[120]

The leader makes sure to connect with everyone they can before anything else, if possible!

---

120 Joko Beck, the first female American Zen Master and a badass at cutting through bullshit. Look her up.

Please try to include everyone in an invitation to go out for some tea, or another nice thing to do for those who would like to connect.

Compassionate Recovery circles can also focus on specific topics such as addictions, principles such as honesty, kindness, forgiveness, and life skills like meditation, yoga, and compassionate communication. There are many possibilities for formats. Groups can focus exclusively on one topic as the theme or change topics based on the community's needs that show up. Your recovery, your way.

Circle of Safety Check-ins

Connect with everyone on your circle of safety team. Bring your journal notes to a meetup with recovery friends. Make it a brunch or a walk, whatever the group feels would enhance life that day. Take turns sharing or asking for support on some of your work with your circle of safety.

Compassionate Creatives

You don't need to be a creative to be creative. Get out there and make something with your recovery community, perhaps for the general community. Here, the idea is to engage the bottom-up, creative part of your internal self-reference point. Or just make stuff. Have fun. Share your work, and its meaning is after the session.

Field Practice: Walk as if you are kissing the earth with your feet.[121]

Get together for a mindful, silent recovery walk in the city or anywhere else that the group feels would be nice. For a more effort-based walk, choose a location that's more on the difficult side of things. Examples would be homeless areas or neighborhoods that are different than your own. Do the gentle, mindful, caring walk in a circle around a room. Give everyone a map of this so they can go at their own pace. No phones, no music. Just mindful presence of all senses, globally. Take in the awareness. Take in the suffering in your inhale. Let it dissolve in your burning Light of Compassion. Exhale your joy. Let the light fill all the beings in your sphere of mindful radiance.

After everyone returns to the starting point, check-in and dedicate the merits.

---

[121] Thich Nhat Hanh (2011). "The Long Road Turns to Joy: A Guide to Walking Meditation", p.90, Parallax Press

Field Practice: Compassionate Service

Weekly, on your own or with your peeps, decide who needs you the most. Then help them. Do this consistently. As an option, try different activities together weekly.

Field Practice: Turn on the Generosity

Do the practice that precedes this one, but an option in generosity. Do this on the fly as you walk to lunch or anywhere else. When you see a homeless person, give them a handful of quarters or dollars. Smile. Look in their eyes. Breathe it in, breathe it out, then move on. Your Compassionate Recovery action is in and out, hit/pass.

Field Practice: Carry the Message

We carry the message of compassion by embodying compassion. We embody it through study, practice, and behavior. This is called heart-min training. The more we train, the better our brain will learn to turn on the healthy switches and circuits. Eventually, we learn how to Drop into compassion. Then we learn to maintain it. Once we maintain compassion long enough to mature, it becomes integrated into our experience.

Collective Practice: Self-compassion

Make a character sketch of three different aspects of yourself. Give each a name. Write about their reason for being. Once you have an idea and a feeling for these parts of you, set aside time for mindful reflection on them. Next, imagine a room familiar to all three components and invite them in. Let them talk to each other. Join the conversation. Ask how they feel. Use compassionate communication.

Following the session, write in your journal in as much detail as possible. Add to it if you wake up at 0300 with something. Don't go back to sleep before jotting it down. Next, buy a gift for each aspect.

Collective Practice: Drop into Calm Patience

We're always waiting for something. In this practice, we sit for an extended period of strict silence and stillness. A minimum time frame would be 45 minutes. During the session, your focus is patience without waiting—practice self-compassion for any challenges. Empathize with the different parts of you.

Let that dissolve as your mind slowly drops to the bottom of a vast, still lake high in the mountains, with pristine white sand at the bottom. Let your mind land softly there, the soundless dust particles floating gently as you rest in your place. Be there, without distraction, until the bell rings.

Extra credit: apply what you learn in your community. Choose the person that requires the most patience. Consider them a gift that will give you the root of your attachment to work on.

Collective Practice: Let the Knot Loosen

Become still. Find your feet. Back straight. Inhale, hold a little open throat, exhale audibly...haaaaa. As you just sit, notice physical knots of tension of any size anywhere in your body, energy, and mind. Be aware of the vibrations of resistance surrounding these knots.

Meditate like this: My ego is a tiny knot in the infinite fabric of the universe. May it loosen, and the wisdom of compassion springs forth. Notice how your pressure on this area increases the tension. Try to intensify it on purpose. Then inhale, let the knot squeeze tight, and exhale as it dissolves into a limp rope. Repeat as necessary as a life practice until you are free of attachment and suffering.

Collective Practice: Day Retreat

Find the time and place to do a personal or group retreat day or half-day. Write up a schedule. Choose the practices that you want to use from this book. Invite people who want to do the work, especially if they don't look like you.

Start and end each session like a Compassion Circle. In a half-day, from 8 am to Noon, do two 90-120 minutes sessions each. Break for lunch—option for silence during mealtime. Dedicate and conclude. For a full day, add a second session from 2 pm-4 pm or make your own schedule. Conclude the retreat with an offering of healthy foods that each person brought. Bless the food and the beings who died so that you could eat.

Write extensively after the retreat for a week or ten days. Allow yourself support for triggers, backdraft, and any funnel traps. Get the support, and stay grounded. This is called integration. It's the main point!

Collective Practice: I Belong Here

Take a moment. Place one or both hands on your face, heart, or belly. Breathe in slowly. Notice how you feel in your body at the moment. Let it settle to the ground between each breath. When you exhale, don't push; only relax and let go.

Let self-compassion seep into your heart, into the core of your being. Allow yourself to be who you are in this moment and know that you belong, right where you are, right now.

Say silently or aloud, "I belong here." Repeat it with a stronger voice. Speak the truth with conviction. Who cares if anyone hears you? You belong here!

Collective Practice: Differentiate

Sensations in our bodies, currents of emotional energy, and difficult thought patterns can result from old traumas. These traumas aren't coherent, logical memories. Experiences happen in fragments that sometimes can seem to be connected to an event but often cannot. This brings about a state of confusion. We wonder why we feel anxiety, helplessness, or anger.

The power of healing can happen when we release the trauma into the now. Sit with your back straight. Come to stillness. If stillness freaks you out as it does for the severely traumatized, you can sway gently in a circle or side to side. If that's too much, take yoga or martial arts, horseback riding, or salsa dancing instead.

Learn to move your body with your breath. Then come back to sitting practice, little by little. Try to integrate movement and stillness.

If you're a sitter, sit still and notice your breath. Be aware of your heartbeat, the rising and falling of your belly—the sensation of air in your nostrils, down the back of your throat. Note what you see, though your eyes are still. See the shadows, the play of light, but let your eyes remain motionless. Notice the feeling of muscles in the back of your eyes. Notice what you hear.

How far away is that sound, where does it come from, and where does it disappear to? Even continuous sounds come in waves.

How is the taste in your mouth? Practice mindful eating when you're eating. But when you're sitting, just notice without moving your tongue. How do you know what you taste while your mouth is still? What do you smell? Don't wrinkle your nose; just notice any scent in the air or your nostrils. Be aware of the changing nature of the sensory experiences in your body. Notice the breath happening the whole time. Thoughts try to penetrate and dominate your awareness. Let them come and go. Label the thought if it helps, a thought about food, a thought about fear. A thought about I don't know what: label and release. Come back to the breath.

The next layer is noticing uncomfortable feelings or sensations, labeling them, or noticing them as not coming from the present moment. This can be a little tricky at times for some of us, but it is, in practice, very simple. Notice a feeling and come back to this present experience.

Notice the difference between what is happening right now and the difficult feelings.

This is key to healing, and if you can do it, even just a little, you'll be amazed at how freeing it is. We might call this a grounding or a present moment meditation, but when we allow our dissociated traumatic feelings to dissolve into the past, and notice that they don't represent the present moment. This is your moment, not the trauma's. Not your perpetrator's.

We can unhook from our trauma. It's a process. It takes diligence and time and patience, and self-compassion. Even if you feel like you can't do it or it's not working, be compassionate to yourself about it. Allow change and growth.

The release comes in the differentiation between now and not now. If you can experience this for even a split second, you can start the process of release. It's important to have support because of backdraft, the response to adding the oxygen of mindfulness to the fuel of past trauma. If it gets overwhelming, stop. Take care of yourself. Get support. Try another type of Compassionate Recovery activity. Come back to this one later. Be kind. Be gentle. But keep going.

It works if you work it. And it won't if you don't.

You wouldn't look through the pages of a cookbook, then complain that the recipe didn't taste good. Bake the cake. Gluten-free and vegan or however you like it.

A little sweat can take you a long way. Just like the gym or learning a language, it's better to do a moderate amount of work consistently than a bunch intermittently. My guitar teacher taught me that 30 minutes a day of concentrated practice is better than 3 hours in a row once a week.

Collective Practice: Consistency

Each person in your group agrees to do the following. After a week, y'all get together and share about it. Make sure someone brings snacks!

Instructions: Copy one practice from this book onto your phone. Commit to doing it every day for five minutes. Make notes each day that you do the practice. If you miss a day, make a note about why. Did something uncomfortable come up? Over a week, you'll know if it's good for you. Next, grab another one and do the same until you have your collection. Remember that your system's collection can be changed and added to whenever you need it to. Be careful not to switch things up too often without getting into some deep areas. Sometimes we tend to move on when things get complicated. Stick with it.

Your journal is a sacred practice. A witch that I had on my podcast told me that witches always keep a book of spells and symbols, notes, and charms. Make your journal magical.

The practices are included to allow everyone of different backgrounds to learn something about themselves. The information here is meant to be practical and to last a long time in your recovery.

Sharing is caring. When we get together and form compassion-based connections with good communication and agreement on a healthy path of recovery, it changes our brain. The good news is that even though the addiction and trauma circuits can't be erased, neither can the self-compassion and others that we're doing here. You build a home to rest safely in.

Collective Practice: Stages of Compassion

- Compassion for self
- Compassion for close friends, family
- Compassion for all the anonymous people
- Compassion for the difficult people
- Compassion for all beings, without exception

These practices can be thought of as stages that go from an aspiration, or a wish, to an actual feeling of compassion. Our actions can be geared towards compassionate acts before we even feel it. We might call this acting as if. Sometimes we begin to feel it only after taking positive actions in that direction. Bring your body; your heart will follow.

Brain research tells us that if we smile, we feel happier. If we don't smile unless we feel like smiling, we don't get that result of cultivating happiness by taking the action of smiling. The same is true for focusing on positive emotions. People who do intentional practice on positive emotions wind up feeling better. This is a pretty important point for those of us in recovery. We don't often feel like being nice or going to work or making amends to someone. But when we take the actions, shifts happen.

Keep in mind that each of the stages of compassion may take a while to develop depending on what comes up for us. Some say that the practice of absolute compassion can take many lifetimes. The point is that all our principles and practices can be cultivated, nurtured, and strengthened. They're dose-related.

Compassion is the glue that holds humanity together. Without it, we would undoubtedly cause more harm to each other and our planet than we already do. For addicts, it's imperative to have a practice that keeps us connected to ourselves and our community. If you have an urge to use your drug of choice, you can do a simple practice of mindful self-compassion that will help keep you sober for that day. You can even write down messages to yourself in advance, such as,

"Hey, I care about you. Stay sober one more day!"

Keep in mind that it's easy to pay lip service to compassion. We think that we understand it because it's talked about so much. It's just a feeling, right? Why do we need to make such a big deal about it? The truth is that while compassion lives within us all, we are mostly out of touch with it. If we were to truly embody compassion, which the Tibetans call absolute *bodhicitta,* Sanskrit for compassion, we would be enlightened beings with compassion even for people who were torturing them, such as in the case of Tibetan monks who were held by the Chinese government.

A being who has realized absolute bodhicitta would put compassion ahead of a threat to physical survival. That's mastery. For us, baby steps!

Is addiction an act of compassion or an act of self-loathing? If you had compassion for yourself, how would you treat yourself regarding your addictions?

Any of the practices in the Stages of Compassion can be done standalone for as many months or years as you like. They can be done in order, or not, as much or as little as they work for you. Don't push. The door opens from the inside.

My recommendation with all practice is that you set a time to do it regularly and consistently. Again, a little bit of work on a consistent basis will yield more results than a lot of practice sporadically. That's how I wrote this book over more than four years!

Tip: You can record the instructions written or use your own words. Play them back during the practice session. Leave space between the sentences. Let the message sink in as much as it does each session. Don't push.

Keep a journal for each one of these practices. Record your feelings after every session. Be sure to date your entries. Share them with your circle of safety. You must go deep into these practices because the wounds are deep in your amygdala and throughout your body.

1. Settle into Stillness

Set your timer for 10 minutes. Sit comfortably with your back straight. You can also use a chair, cushion, or the floor with your legs cross-legged, half cross-legged, or folded under you. Allow your body to become still. Commit to being still for the whole 10 minutes, no matter what. No itching or scratching. No Tik-Tok.

Be still. Let yourself feel your body as it is for the whole time you've committed to it. If you forget to be still, bring yourself back gently to stillness.

2. Self-compassion

After settling in, reflect on everything that you've been through. How is your body feeling? Is it light, heavy, soft, or firm? Where is there unease, tension, or distress? Notice your suffering. If you feel fine, just notice that you are in your body and be grounded. Your body was born, has grown up, and will grow older. This is the reality for everyone. It's impermanent, like all phenomena. Notice what the meditation brings up for you. During this practice, or whenever you need to, put one or both hands on your chest, or your face and say, "May I be at ease." Repeat this six times as a lotus petal opens from the center, one petal at a time, until the lotus of compassion is in full bloom. Sit in the radiance of that bloom.

From that position, imagine another person that is like you but suffering more. In your meditation, practice giving your joy and goodness to that person on the exhale. When you inhale, take all their sufferings in as dark smoke that dissolves into the rainbow-colored lotus at your heart.

3. Friends and Family Compassion Plan

Do the practice of opening to stillness for 20 minutes—option to do the preceding practices. Then recall someone close to you. It's best not to begin with anyone very challenging for you. Start easy. Take your time. Consider their path in life. How have they struggled? What were the challenges that they faced? Meditate on one thing that has caused them suffering. Can you empathize? If it's a struggle, let yourself settle back to stillness. How have you experienced their suffering? Have you taken on their distress? Can you discriminate the difference? What did you see? How did it affect you? How does it make you feel when you consider the suffering that they've experienced? Notice where in your body you feel the experience of being aware of their suffering. Hold that space for yourself and them. Just sit mindfully for a while without trying to fix your feelings or analyze how you can help them or give them advice.

To cultivate compassion, bring about the wish they be free of suffering. This is the aspiration level of compassion. You are developing it with this practice. Cultivate the awareness of the other person's suffering and bring forward the wish that they are free of suffering. Say the words, "May they be free of suffering." Once more, with feeling.

You'll notice it's easy to cultivate compassion for someone that you already love. That's why we start there, so you can get used to the feeling and bringing up compassion as an intentional practice in a way that's attainable and sets us up for success.

Next, make an action plan for how you will do things that benefit the ones closest to you because you can. They're right there.

4. Compassion for Strangers

Begin with a 35-minute settling into stillness. This goes deeper into the wisdom of stillness that evokes more global compassion beyond our usual boundaries. Notice how stillness supports your practice. Sink into it, but don't fall asleep. If you feel sleepy, look up a little. If you feel agitated, look down a little. If you're chill as a mf, look straight on, baby.

Consider the previous meditations on compassion for yourself and a loved one. It's time to cultivate the feeling of caring, of wanting the people around your community that you see but are otherwise strangers to you. Cultivate the authentic wish for this person to not suffer. Feel it in your bones. If you begin to feel triggered or distressed, return to stillness. Stay in it, don't end sessions early.

Reflect on one stranger at first, one whose name you don't know. If you're out and about, look in the face of one stranger. Try to take an energetic snapshot of them to use in your meditation. Imagine their soul. What do they want? Is it different from you? How do you think they experience suffering? Cultivate the wish for them to be at ease by saying, "May this stranger be at ease. May they be free of suffering."

Allow the feeling of compassion to arise within you. If there's a knot of resistance, hold it in your palm with warm compassion. If you have no sense of that desire to end suffering today, return to the first practice and start there. It will vary for you at different times. It's different for everyone. Let it be fluid for you.

Compassion for the anonymous, nameless, faceless people of the world is harder sometimes and often easier for those we don't know anything about. But can you imagine that every one of the people you don't know shares the common humanity of suffering? Do you feel that they want to be free of suffering, just like you, and just like those you love? Can you develop the wish that they, too, can be at ease and free from suffering? If this is too hard, work on developing the desire to wish. There is no wrong starting point. As with everything in this book, start where you are. Your recovery, your way.

5. Anonymous Compassion

Be still for 35 minutes. Review the previous practices slowly, one by one, in as much energetic-emotional feelings as you can muster. Let it well up but stay regulated within your current window of tolerance. Compassion is already who you are. It's who they are, too, even if we have no idea or sense of the billions of anonymous humans on the planet, living and dying every moment without end. Everyone is part of the sea of bodies in a busy train station or airport. This kind of anonymous compassion warms you like a lovely blanket. Imagine that nice blanket of compassion laying gently across the wounds of the oceans of people. Send the light from your rainbow radiant lotus heart right into their hearts. Breathe in their darkness.

Breathe out your light. Do this twenty-one times. Use a mala or prayer beads to count.

Return to stillness practice for five to ten minutes.

6. Compassion for the Evildoers

Sit for 35 minutes in silent awareness. If you're going to intellectualize this, please return to square one instead. You'll be way ahead of the game if you can get a taste of a few moments of it. A little compassion on any of these levels is like a hot spring in the middle of a forest. Sink in. Learn to savor it. Self, loved one, stranger, anonymous ocean of people, slowly. Notice what is the same about your experience of compassion for each of those. What changes? Is it your willingness to be present with your own feelings, or judgments about the others?

Think about a person who has caused great harm to you or anyone else. Don't try to do this meditation on the biggest, grossest bad actions or actors. Make a list of some and pick somebody lower on the intensity scale, to begin with. Try that. This isn't an all at once practice. It's a life practice. It takes time and effort. Or maybe non-effort is a better way to put it. My old teacher used to say, "Being just this moment, compassion's way." Feel free to add to or subtract from your list. Compassion is patient. Do your best. Even just wishing to be willing is a beginning. Why? Because it will open the magic in your heart and help keep you connected to the world and part of the community, and it will support your agency to choose who you want to be in this life.

Keep your breath regulated so you can stay regulated. You don't have to do this. Feel free to pause at any time. The opportunity is yours when you decide to return to the most festering wound. To continue, practice compassion for the bad players in our world is a spiritual act. There's no way to bypass here and be legit at the same time. You're going to heal as deep as you're going to heal. Be aware of spirals and funnels. Remember your brain circuitries. This is burning a new one that will support your freedom from these bonds of suffering. Do the practice. Stay in it. Stay with your breath. Notice the body.

What kind of ACEs did this person possibly experience? They must have been lonely and terrified when they experienced atrocities on innocent victims. Surely it would be insane to consider anything but wrath for them. But here we are. The development of compassion matters most right here, in the realm where we want to practice it the least.

You might think, would Jesus or Buddha or another spiritual figure have compassion for even the least among us? It's said that they did. But we will have our doubts.

We're not that holy.

Those people don't deserve compassion.

They did this. They did that.

But the aspiration of compassion doesn't require that you feel it all for everyone all at once. The Light of Compassion already exists within you. It knows no bounds. Did your addiction have bounds? Be real. Let your recovery progress with your brain neurology into a new mind space of good vibes.

Compassion is partly the feeling of noticing the suffering of another and cultivating the wish that it would go away. You're not taking any physical actions right now. At this moment, you are safe.

Are you willing to be willing to consider that?

Extra credit: write this out and work on it over time with the awareness that it is a process. There is no rush.

7. Compassion for All Beings

Sit in deep silent awareness for 35 minutes. This is the final stage of all compassion training. But don't feel that you have to graduate. Listen well to your own heart. Feel as profoundly as you can the previous meditations on compassion. How is it, just now? How is your breathing? What is the feeling at your heart center? Is your body heavy or light, depressed or energized? Where are you in your window of tolerance? Be aware and rest in stillness like a newborn baby. All the unresolved psychological attachments that we have can be released here. It's up to you.

Return to that feeling of warmth and compassion at the heart center. The endless, still space in which we dwell holds infinite trillions of numberless millions of conscious beings that feel pain, who come into being in places that we see and do not see. They live and grow old and suffer and die. The Sanskrit term for this realm is samsara. We are all in the same boat.

There's no way to have time to consider an infinite number of beings. We can bring up a few and cultivate compassionate intentions for them as they arise. But then, at some point, we can make our wish for all beings to be at ease, free of suffering. You may put your palms together at the heart center and say, "May all beings be free of suffering." Savor the moment. Let it rise and swell within you.

Extra credit: Throughout the days, come back to this aspiration as often as possible, and cultivate the aspiration by creating a new circuit in your brain with the words,

May all beings be free of suffering.

May all beings enjoy perfect comfort and ease.

That is the practice[122]. However, many times we forget or become distracted, we bring ourselves back to mindful compassion.

Take the feelings from all these practices into your community, where they need your compassion.

---

[122] Extra-extra credit: Refrain from total liberation from suffering until the infinite oceans of numberless beings of all kinds, tiny and massive, are relaxed and happy, sitting in a pool of comfort and ease. Just like you want for yourself.

Notes

Conclusion

The strongest attachment for any of us is to the ego. Surrender without inflation or spiritual bypassing is the practice that collapses the ego. That can be scary. But if we've done the work to regulate our stress responses and maintain mindful, self-compassionate focus with patience and an attitude of generosity, we will step forward on our journey from attachment-addiction to recovery-mastery as if our feet are kissing the Earth.

We devote ourselves to compassionate service to others to free ourselves and them from suffering. But if we have high ACEs, I want to make one last point. The practice doesn't ask you to succumb to victimization or abuse in a distorted attempt at service. You will keep your self-compassionate self-empowerment as you work to help others. The days of cowering to do our perp's bidding are never to be repeated. We're healing now. Keep that attitude, and I'm confident that you'll do fine.

Bless you, for reading this book. It's the way I see things. After all these years of study and reflection, I'm still trying to move my feet to help others. Hopefully, this book is a helpful step for you on your roadmap of recovery. There is a lot of content to the story. I tried to write it in a way that hits home for the people who need it most. As I said, this book responds to what I've learned from you, my kind readers. You are my community.

Thank you for being willing to get raw and do the work. It is the next step in our evolution toward mastery. We must evolve or perish. You're an important part of the healing, so thank you.

I hope that as addicts with ACEs, or wherever we are on the spectrum, we will evolve beyond suffering to a life of comfort and ease.

We are all Lights of Compassion. May we shine our radiant light everywhere it is needed, for every being who needs it, for as long as necessary.

Additional Resources

Compassion Cultivation Training
www.compassioninstitute.com
Mindful Self Compassion
www.selfcompassion.org
National Child Traumatic Stress Network
www.nctsn.org
Internal Family Systems
www.selfleadership.org
Dialectical Behavioral Therapy
www.pdbti.org
ACEs in Urban Populations
https://www.philadelphiaaces.org

What's Next

There is ongoing research that will no doubt add to the Compassionate Recovery database. For that reason, it will be necessary to update this book at regular intervals. Expect it. In addition to updates and revisions based on your feedback@compassionaterecovery.us, many chapters and topics were left on the cutting room floor. Some of those will go up on the website or be used for a possible video series. New ideas can be added to follow-up volumes, such as a workbook. There would be space to focus on some of the work of Compassionate Recovery in more detail than was possible in one broad-reaching volume.

With new ideas forthcoming, there are many possibilities, so please stay tuned. Join us at http://compassionaterecovery.us

In terms of community, this is entirely up to you. Take this book with you and find like-minded souls to go over some of the materials with a small group. If there is a need and interest in building a compassionate community, there certainly continues to be a need for solutions to the problems of trauma and addictions. If you have questions or need support, contact the author directly at info@compassionaterecovery.us

If you found this book helpful, please leave an honest review on Amazon. It helps get the word out!

Books for Addicts

Many for whom this book was written need your help to get it into their hands and find the power of compassion to heal addictions. On the site, you can
- Send books to
  - Treatment center clients
  - Correctional Facilities
  - Community Programs
  - Churches
- Your book(s) can be sent anonymously if you wish
- Sign up for mentorship of someone in need of support.
- Be listed as a resource.

For more, visit http://compassionaterecovery.us

About the Author

Darren Littlejohn graduated with an associate degree in Behavioral Science from San Jose City College, obtained a Bachelor of Arts in Psychology from California State University, and completed all coursework, no thesis, for a master's degree in Research Psychology.

As a certified power yoga instructor, he's taught since 2011 in gyms and studios along the West Coast. For many years following the release of the bestselling book, *The 12-Step Buddhist* (Atria\Beyond Words 2009, 2018), Darren led workshops and retreats in the Pacific Northwest. This is his tenth title.

Darren Littlejohn's Amazon Author Profile
https://www.amazon.com/author/darrenlittlejohn

Twitter @12stepbuddhist
Instagram @12stepbuddhist
The 12-Step Buddhist Podcast can be found on Spotify, iTunes, Youtube, and https://the12stepbuddhist.libsyn.com

Made in the USA
Coppell, TX
29 May 2022